The place I'm in

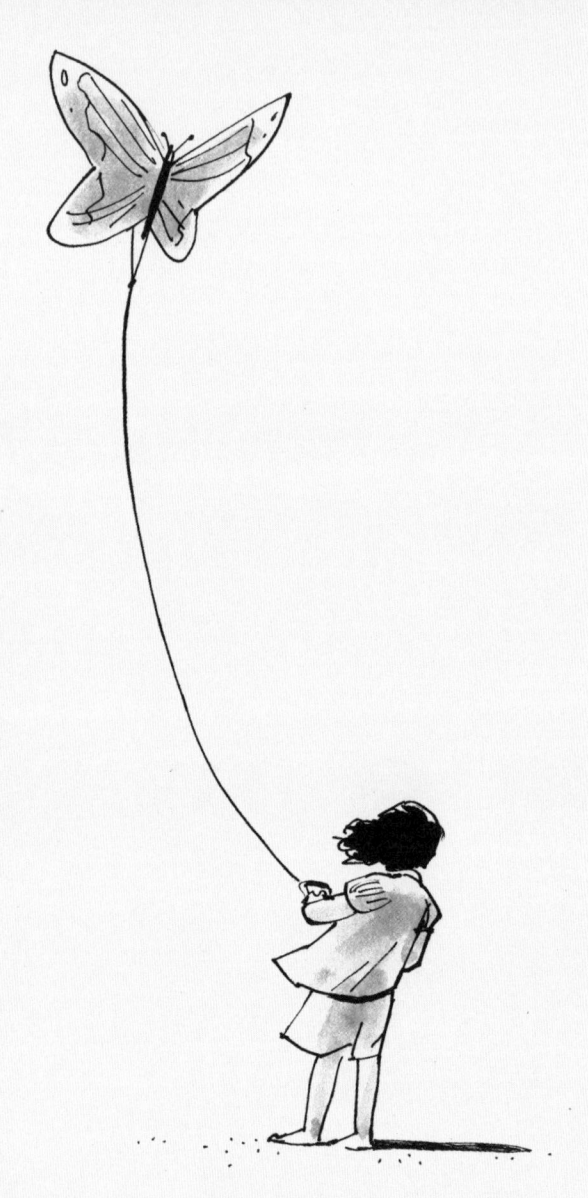

To Bea and Duncan, who fill my heart with joy.

Miranda Keeling
Illustrations by Adam Beer

The place I'm in
WHAT I SEE WHEN I STOP TO NOTICE

Leaping Hare Press

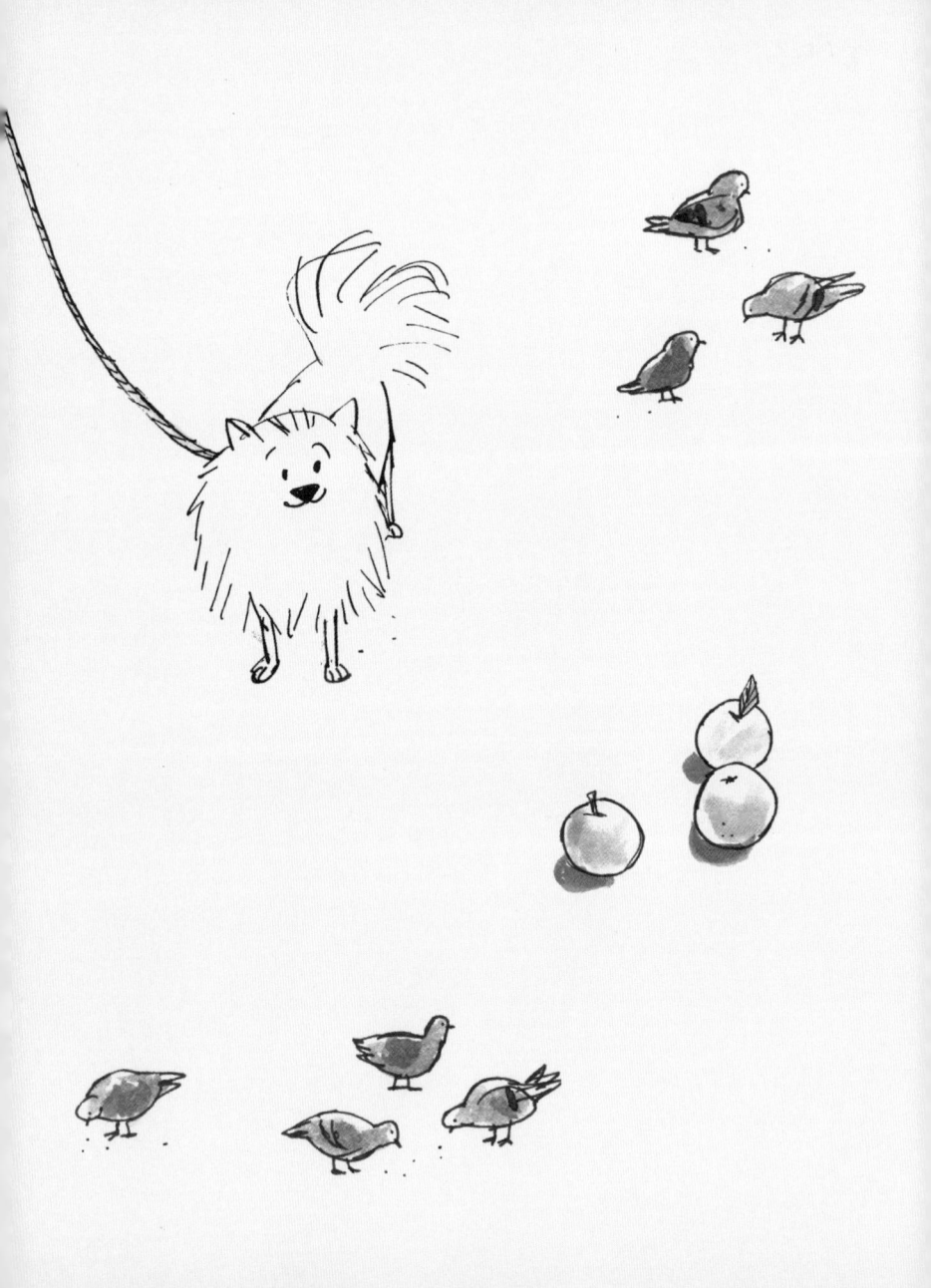

CONTENTS

6   Introduction

8   ● Setting out
26   ● At the park
42   ● In a café
60   ● On the street
78   ● Popping in
96   ● In the countryside
114   ● At the seaside
132   ● On the move
150   ● Nightlife
168   ● Coming home

189   Acknowledgements
190   About the author/About the illustrator

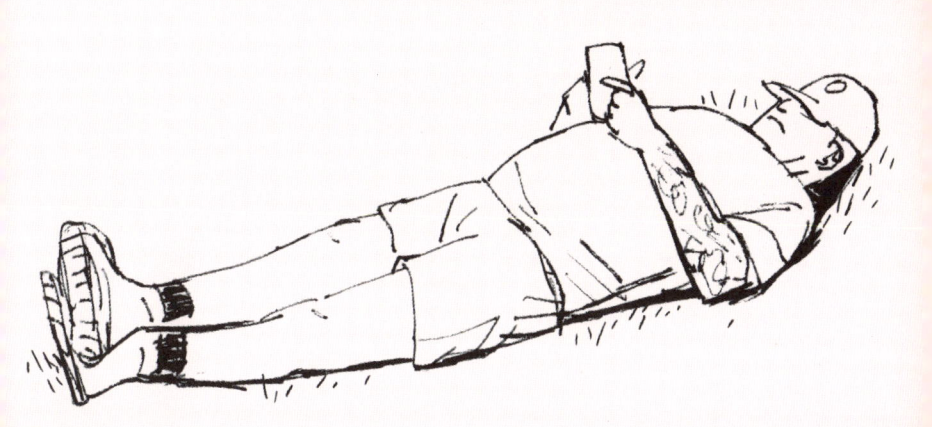

INTRODUCTION

Most of the things that make up my day will be familiar to you. I wake up in the morning. I leave the house to go to work or to do something else. I walk or cycle or take the bus or the train. I don't drive; perhaps you do. I go to the supermarket. I queue at the post office.

    I sit in a café. I notice a man opposite me in a brown knitted hat. He folds a receipt from his pocket into the shape of a boat and places it on the white sea of his plate as he gets up to leave. I walk down the street. I notice the buildings reflected in puddles from the recent rain. A breeze blurs the bricks. I collect a parcel from my local corner shop. Outside, a dog in a yellow padded coat whines for her owner.

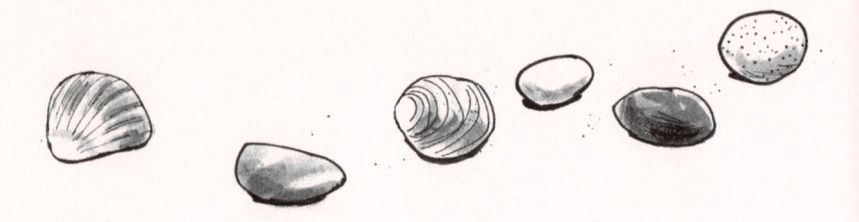

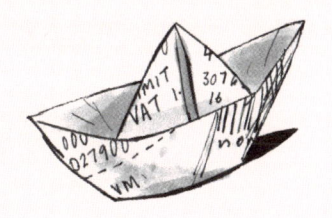

I walk through an old part of the city. I feel cobbles under my feet. I see a single cloud in the clear sky. More clouds form, and now the sky is full and dark. I close my eyes against the sleet.

I collect these moments like people collect pebbles and shells in their pockets at the seaside. Maybe they'll take them home and put them in the bathroom or maybe they'll tip them back onto the sand before they go. The moments around me are all real and tangible, whether I stop to notice them or not, or whether I carry them with me or leave them on the shore.

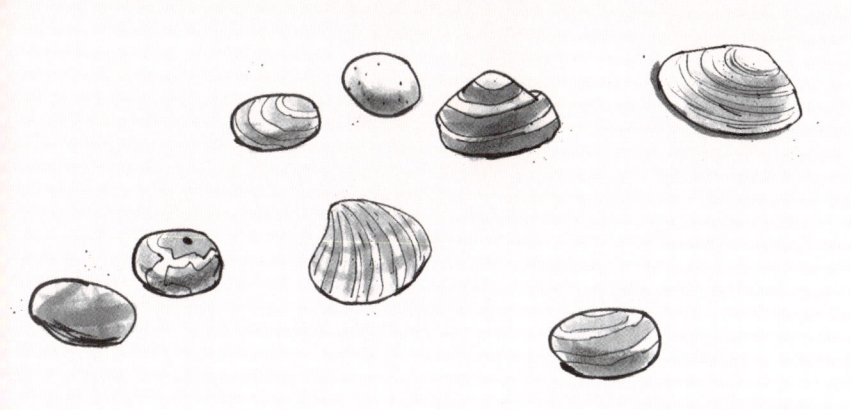

SETTING OUT

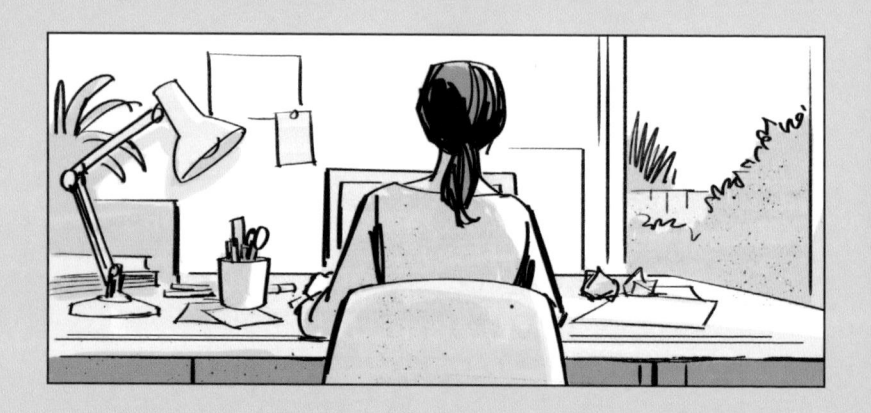

I move a scrunched-up receipt to the left of the pens on my desk. They were on the right – literally a displacement activity. I look through the glass desktop at my foot. My sandals are comfortable and old. The leather is cracked at the sides. They will need replacing soon. Noticing in my home brings with it the usual, endless to-do lists: things to sort, fix, sell, clean, put away, give away, throw away – like a repetitive list in one of my daughter's Dr Seuss books.

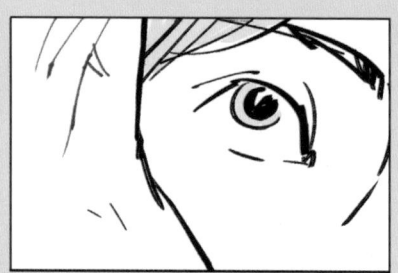

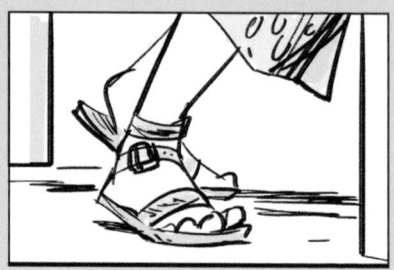

An aeroplane goes overhead, its noise cutting across the wind in the trees. My door is open to the garden. I have so much to do there.

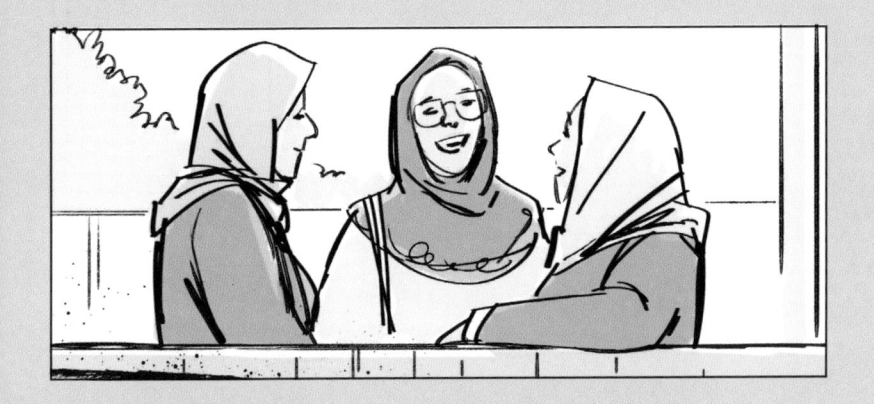

In order to calm the list hum, I look out at the sky or listen to my neighbours talking on the street. Or I zoom in to the curved edge of my computer keyboard. But the edge is chipped. And one of the keys is a bit stuck. I must do something about that.

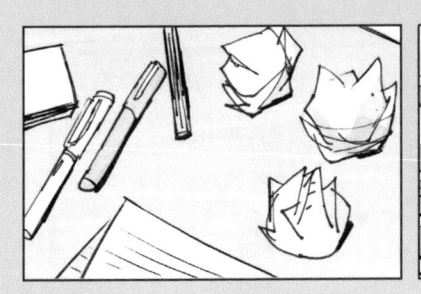

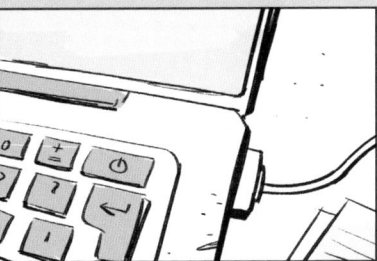

I hear my doorbell. There is a little boy
standing at my front door.
Little boy: I live in the house behind you.
Me: Ah. Hello.
Little boy: Your tree has three apples left. I
can see from my garden. Can I pick them?
Me: Can you do it safely?
Little boy: Yes.
Me: Then sure. Thank you for asking.
Little boy: Thank you for the apples.

In the middle of a busy day working at the kitchen table, I notice my cat simply sitting and closing her eyes to the sound of the rain on the roof and so I do the same.

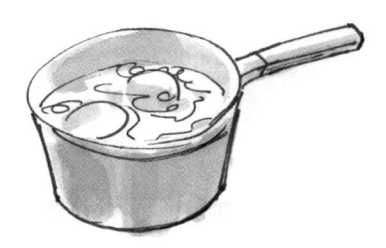

Eggs boil in my pan with a rumbly, clunking sound. The voices of the couple next door float over the fence – they are distorted by the distance, like the voices of the grown-ups in a *Peanuts* cartoon.

A man jogs past the window. He wears a white t-shirt and on it an image of a screaming wolf-teeth bared, its mouth dark red.

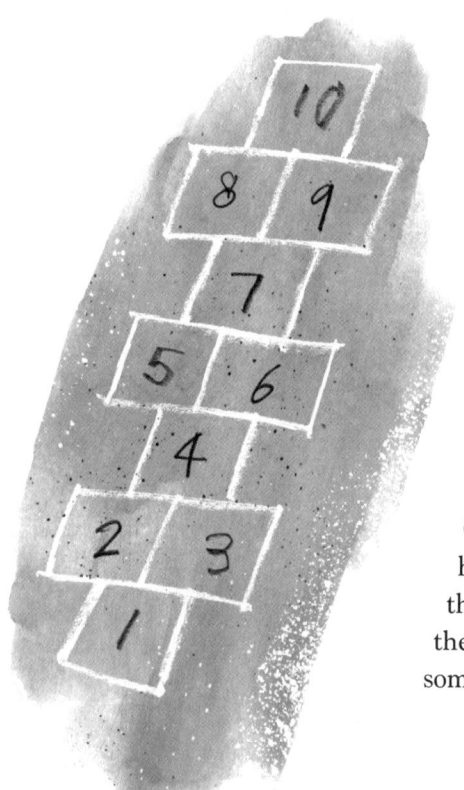

Leaving my house earlier than usual, I see the city that I normally sleep through. A man delivers milk to a dark doorstep. We mumble good mornings. A Deliveroo cyclist arrives home from a late shift, taking off his large, square backpack at the door with a small sigh.

Children have been playing hopscotch outside my front gate, their chalk markings decorating the pavement, and I love it that some things never change.

As I observe the morning sun and post it online, a follower on the other side of the world thanks me for sending the sunlight. It is midnight where she is.

The place I'm in

In the early light, shadows stretch far across the tarmac. A man leans back into his chair in a café. He watches another man walk past the window carrying oranges in orange plastic netting. Their waxy sides are shining.

Mum on the school run: Ready, spaghetti?
Little boy: Just ready.
Mum: Oh, you've grown out of 'Ready, spaghetti'?
Little boy: Not completely.
Just this morning.

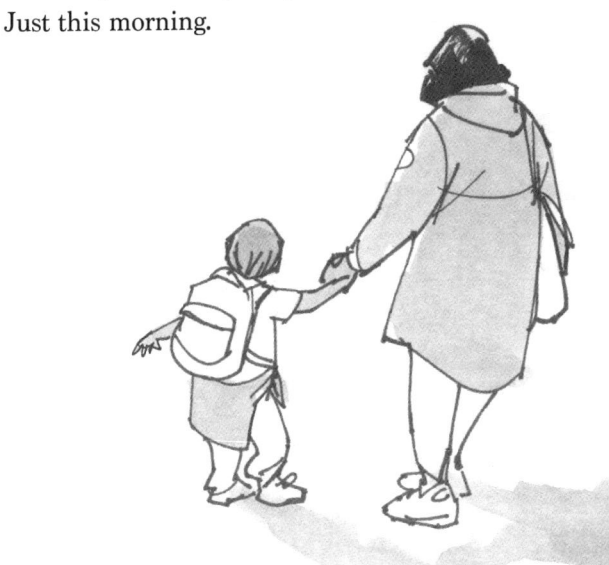

I walk past a familiar coffee shop a bit later
than I usually do. The woman inside who is
normally arranging chairs has finished and is
leaning against the counter, sipping her own
coffee as she blinks at the day.

Teenagers behind me as they walk to college
discuss English lessons. One of them is
struggling with story-writing.
His friend: Just put your feelings in, bruv.
That's the heart of it.

I walk past three women on my route. They
are always on the same corner. Every day a
small difference – the colours of their hijabs,
the atmosphere. Today they discuss something
serious. Yesterday they were leaning on each
other with laughter. It is comforting.

A man sits on a bench in his front garden.
He has three blue stars tattooed on each arm.
He smiles at me through the steam rising
from his cup of tea.

> Men load rubbish from a front garden into
> a van. Rusty barbed wire snakes over an old,
> wooden fence. Up above, telephone wires
> dissect the sky.

I wonder what on earth the local
schoolchildren are up to this morning,
until I realize what they're all carefully
searching for ... conkers.

Monday hangs around. A woman waits for a
bus, a plastic bag tied round her hair, perhaps
ready for rain. A small boy avoids cracks in the
pavement in his glittery jelly shoes.

A mechanic in an empty garage in Hackney
dances his polishing cloth through the air to
classical music, as the sun streams in.

Through the early-morning mist, a vacuum
cleaner by a window becomes a swan accepting
bread with a graceful tilt of its white, plastic neck.

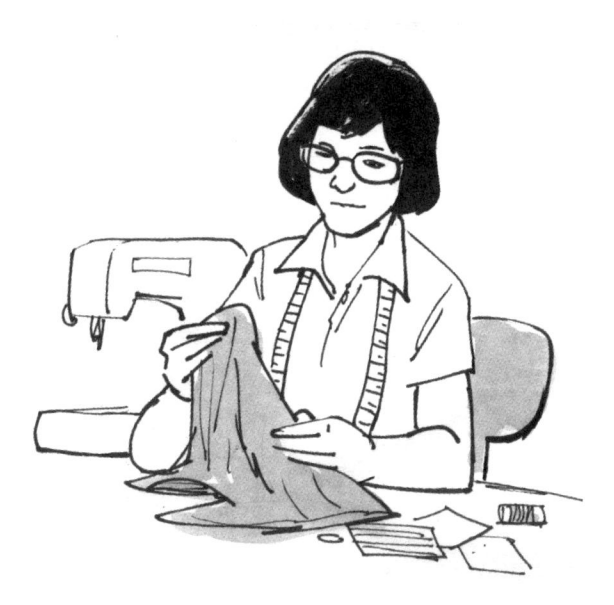

A woman sits at the window of a dry
cleaner with an unfurled tape measure
worn like a scarf. She concentrates on a
blue dress she is mending.

> A gigantic, grey tarpaulin, half
> enveloping a motorbike, flaps noisily
> in the wind like a great bird of prey.

A boy ambushes his little brother on the way
to school, hiding badly on purpose so they
both collapse laughing when he jumps out.

Paint spilled on the pavement becomes a face,
features stretched wide in a quiet, frozen cry.

>From the open window of a terraced house,
a cat leans out and sharpens its claws on
the pebble dash.

A round, sweaty man jogs in a
red and gold tracksuit, his mouth
opening and closing like a fish.

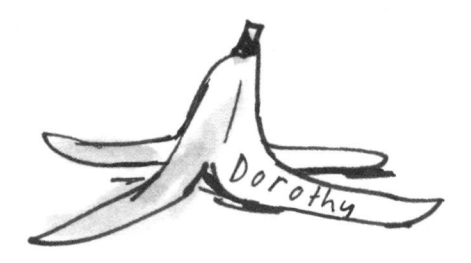

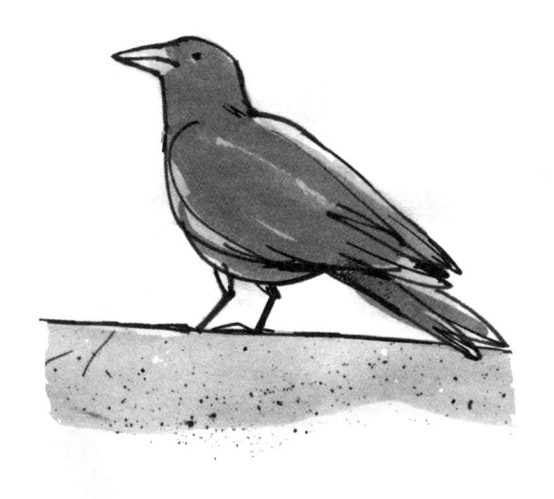

In the new light of just-spring, a banana
skin rests on a quiet street, one word
carefully scratched into its soft, yellow
side: 'Dorothy'.

A crow on a wall caws at a woman
nearby. She stops and mutters
something. It tips its head in a little
nod at her, and flies off.

At the window of a house in Hackney,
above a row of ancient, faded, plastic
orchids, an out-of-season Santa sits on a
bed of silver tinsel.

                    Over a billboard outside a church that says,
                    'Jesus is the only way', someone has carefully
                    balanced a local minicab leaflet.

Little girl watering a front garden in north
London with her mum: Oh no, only one
sunflower has come up.
Her mum: One's better than none, my love.

A woman with a peroxide blonde
mohican has a pink skeleton painted
on her leather jacket, like she's in some
kind of punk x-ray machine.

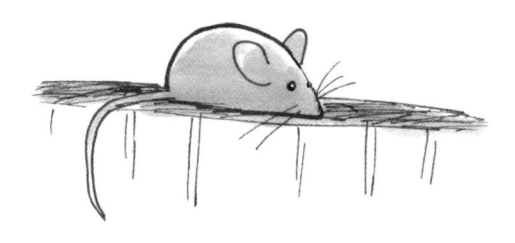

Beside a recycling bin in town, a red-faced man
places a small, brown, wooden mouse. He gives
it a final pat as if to say, 'Good luck, mate.'

My water bottle has leaked in my bag. Inside, the
water has done entrancingly tidal things with the
purple-inked observations in my notebook.

Three clear plastic bags float through the
grey-white sky on the high road, delicately
opening and closing in the wind like
urban jellyfish.

A black-and-white cat on a doorstep
shows her general approval at the
world in a series of long,
slow blinks.

Inside the dim interior of the butcher's
shop, my local butcher sharpens his
knives. He nods me a cheerful
'hello' as I peer in.

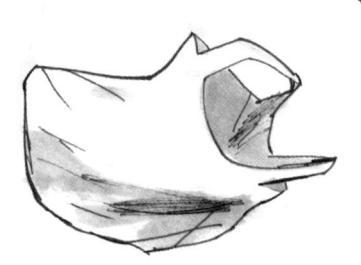

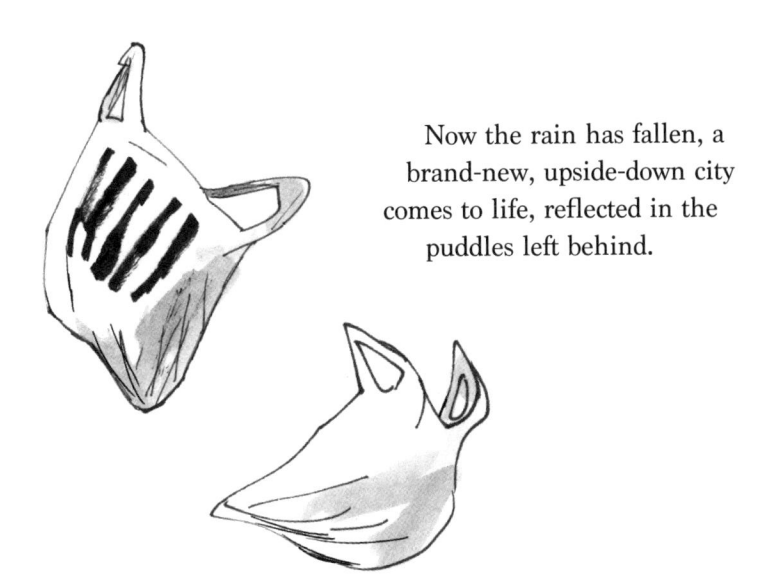

Now the rain has fallen, a brand-new, upside-down city comes to life, reflected in the puddles left behind.

Man in a newsagent: Oh, you know what it's like – when it's cold we complain it's cold, when it's hot we complain it's hot.

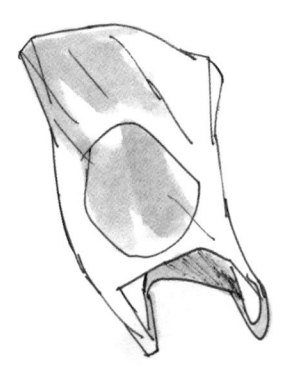

The shadow of a leafy tree falls across a car, the pattern breathtaking in its constantly moving complexity.

Setting out 23

There is a shop I pass on my morning walk that sells handles. That is all it sells. Every morning, the same man is sitting in the empty shop, polishing them. Each time, I feel like I can read an emotion on his face. Today he seems on the edge of melancholy, but his cup of tea is helping.

Autumn leaves blow in the breeze, all yellow-gold and deep rust, and I feel the first cold fingers of the coming winter stroke my bare skin.

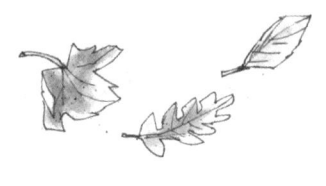

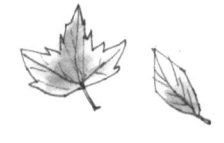

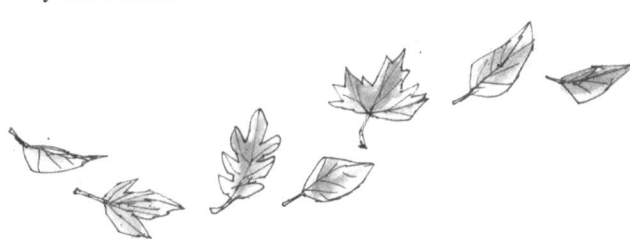

A man looks out of an office window at the rain.
He scowls. Behind him on the wall is taped a
poster printed with the word, 'Optimism'.

> At the window of a house in East London, a carved
> horse's head, with ears pricked up, contemplates
> the book-filled room with pale, wooden eyes.

With an almighty crash, a vast, metal bin outside
Tesco loses its wrestling match against the
wind and falls onto the road.

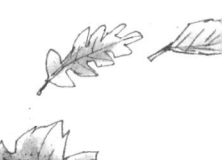

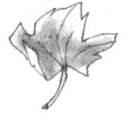

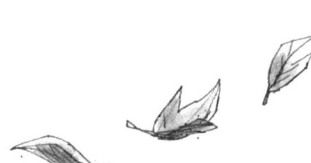

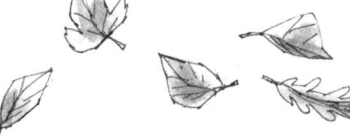

> Little boy in Hackney: Where are we going?
> His dad: School.
> Little boy: Oh.
> [Pause]
> Dad: Where would you like to go?
> Little boy: Barbados.

Setting out

AT THE PARK

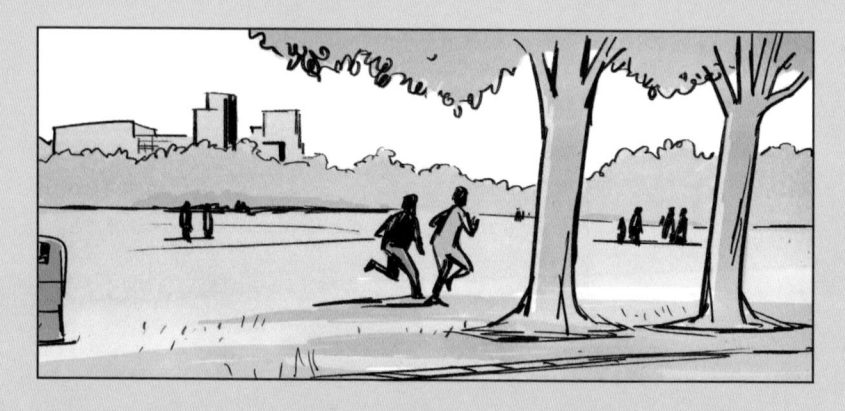

If there's a chance to walk through a park, I'll take it, unless it's late at night. I enjoy looking further into the distance or listening to the wind in the leaves of a large tree. Especially a poplar – something about the shape and arrangement of its leaves makes it sound like the sea.

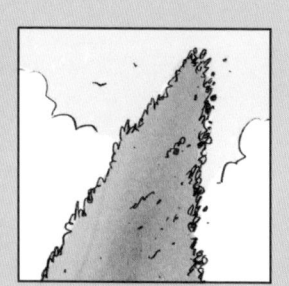

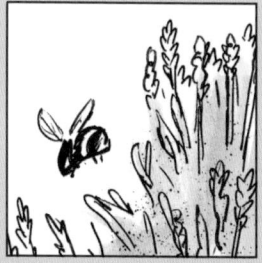

I live in a city full of the great whoosh of trains and buses and cars, so I crave things that move in a natural way – the grass fluttering, birds swooping, a bee diligently making its way around a lavender bush. It's how I cope with the roar of London and the roar of thoughts in my mind. I pick up my 'park pebbles' whenever I find myself in one.

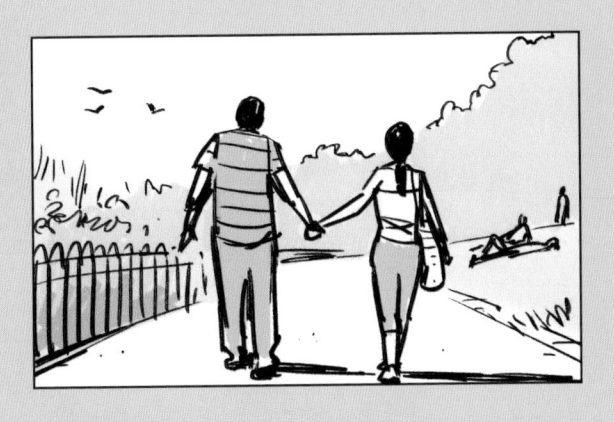

People are fascinating and familiar here. They bring picnics, books, dogs, frisbees, footballs, bunting and a circus kit. They come to bake in the sun or to think, to talk privately on the phone or to a friend or with a group to celebrate a birthday. They stay for a while or cycle through. Sometimes it's calm and beautiful, but also edgy or a place to feel sad or lonely. It's a space we can go without buying a coffee or knowing a code – without a ticket to get in. Our shared gardens.

A woman at the entrance talks to her dachshund, who is refusing to go in, 'You like it when you get there though, don't you?'

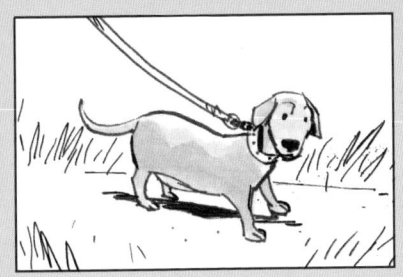

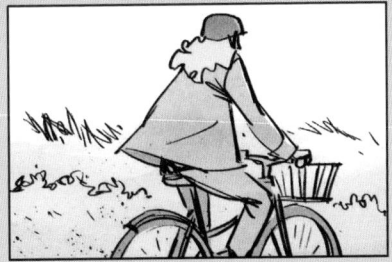

The park is damp and quiet. Leafless
trees sway in the breeze.

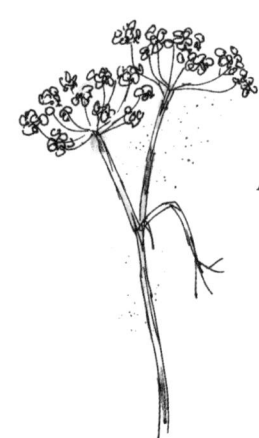

A man sits alone on a bench
in the dark, face shadowed
and hands pressed together
in seeming prayer.

A little girl sees a worm languishing
in the middle of the pavement.
She carries it to some nearby grass,
whereupon it works its way down
into the soft ground.

28 ● **The place I'm in**

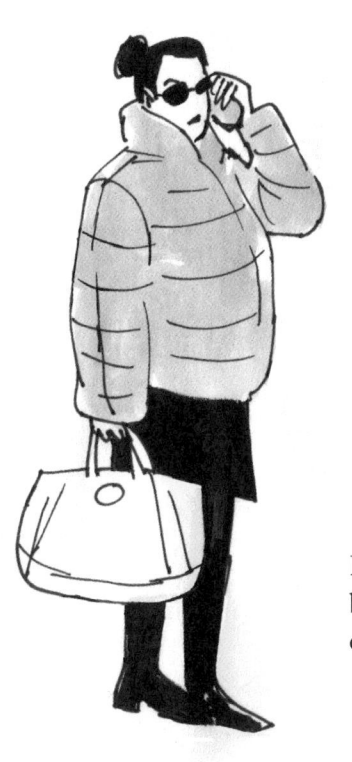

Woman on her phone: Ten minutes. Ten minutes' walk in the park. I'm sure the stationery cupboard will cope, Adeeba.

Pre-teens traverse a skate park – boards swooshing and slamming on the concrete.

The weather turns. Twilight paints the sky purple-grey. Rain pours down in enthusiastic torrents. The cobblestones are dark with it. Bright, urban-wild parakeets fly through the end of summer.

At the park

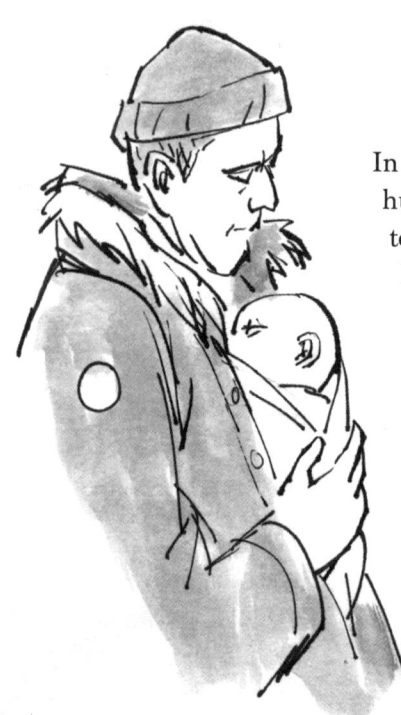

In the crisp cold, a man
hugs a tiny baby in a sling
to his parka-coated chest.
He looks ahead with
sleepy, new-dad eyes.

Through the grey rain, a woman in
a green coat walks a rust-coloured dog.
She stops to pick a snowdrop and places
it behind her ear.

30 ● The place I'm in

This morning, the moon is still
visible in the sky as the sun rises
from behind the trees. I come
across an almost-bear – belly and
legs intact, head and arms gone –
with morning frost still nestling
in its soft-toy fur.

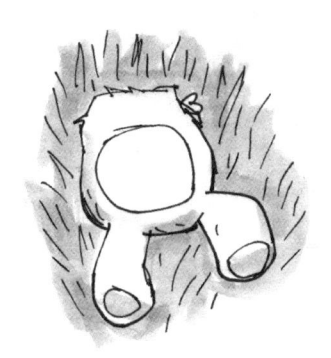

A woman practises boxing, swinging her
gloved fists at the pads held by her trainer.
She is quick and strong and her ponytail
swishes as she weaves and strikes.

I exchange a smile with the mum of a little
boy as a large, brown leaf comes to land at
his feet and he says to it: Are you ok?

A couple stand staring at a lone coot
who has walked out of the water on
his wonderfully big feet and now
eyeballs them back.

Wind, invisible until it moves the trees, causes
the leaves to rustle-whisper. My back is warmed
by the October sun. My daughter has made
friends with another little girl in the playground.
They are already running a busy pizza restaurant.
Things move quickly when you're four.

> Autumn leaves dapple the grass as a little
> boy shouts with joy at the feeling of being
> pushed on a swing.

A woman films her black dog running
through the snow.

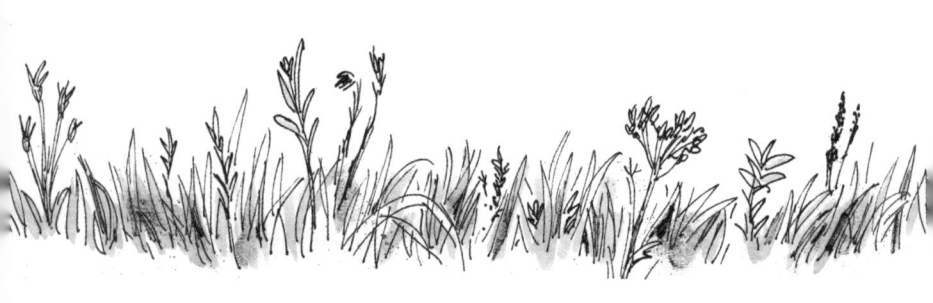

Two women practise Tai Chi pushing hands,
the flowing energy moving back and forth
between them.

A man rollerblades backwards. His hip
movements make a little boy nearby
collapse into giggles.

A small boy in bright blue boots charges
through puddles with a joyous roar.

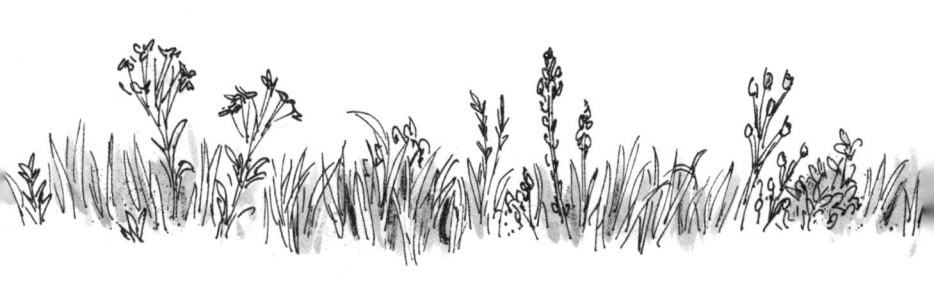

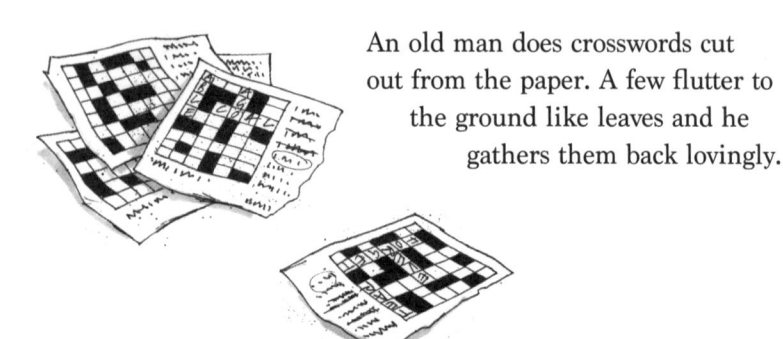

An old man does crosswords cut
out from the paper. A few flutter to
the ground like leaves and he
gathers them back lovingly.

A man in the park talks to his elderly
mother with big, rapid hand gestures and
whatever he is saying makes her smile.

A little girl reads a book as she walks behind her
dad. Suddenly, as if affected by the words on a
page, she sinks down onto the grass and settles in.
A metal cat on a chain around her neck reflects
the last of today's sun.

As the day fades, a woman's shadow follows her faithfully across the park.

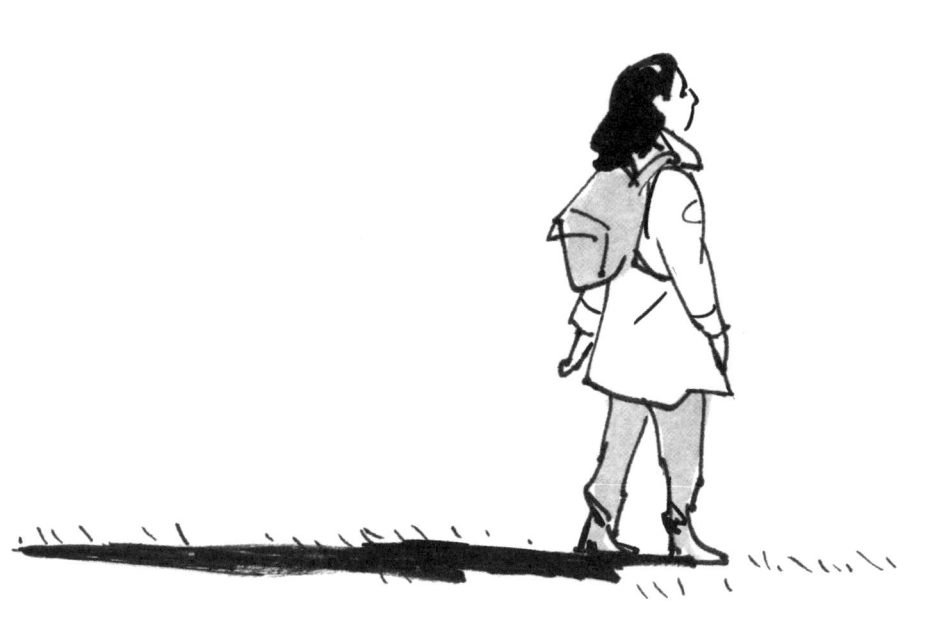

Teenager in the park: There are bare ladybirds
out today; what is this?

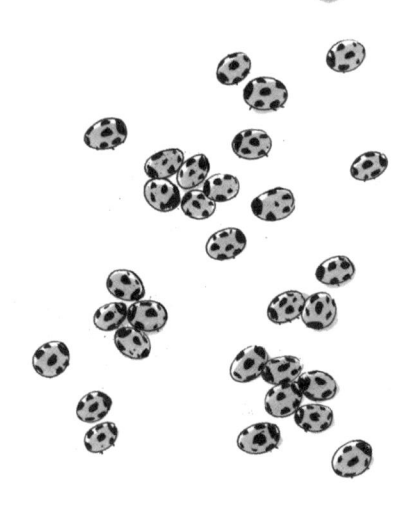

A long-limbed woman in a tango-orange
tracksuit jogs whilst simultaneously removing
her nose ring and putting in a new one.

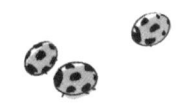

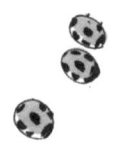

A little girl in a blue coat flashes me
a proud smile as she cycles past, her dad
having finally let go of her bicycle.

A little boy who was running falls over on the grass.
His dad: I told you to be careful!
Boy: It was part of a dance move, actually.

A woman drops her bag and
bends to pick it up, only to
have her glasses fall off her head.
Like a film of my life.

In the middle of a playing field, a
lone metal doorbell rests face-up.
As if to summon someone from
the earth below.

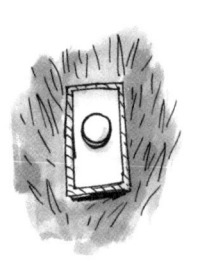

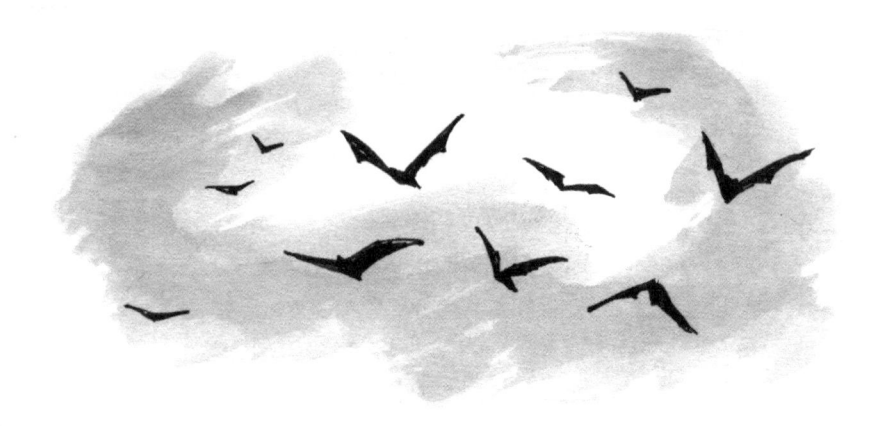

In the park, bats flit around against
a summer solstice sky.

A couple laugh when they find themselves
singing the *Mission Impossible* music together as
they strap their toddler into her pram.

Little girl watching people play on the tennis courts:
They must be trapped in there.

Little girl in the park: I go to ballet today, and tap tomorrow.
Her friend: When do you climb trees?

A little boy sighs as he realizes his mother decided to look the other way just as he finally managed to do a perfect cartwheel.

A woman asks me to take her photo. She wears a green and gold dress and a graduation gown and cap. I take her photo. I ask her what her subject is and she says, 'Cognitive and Computational Neuroscience'. Her pride paints a smile across us both.

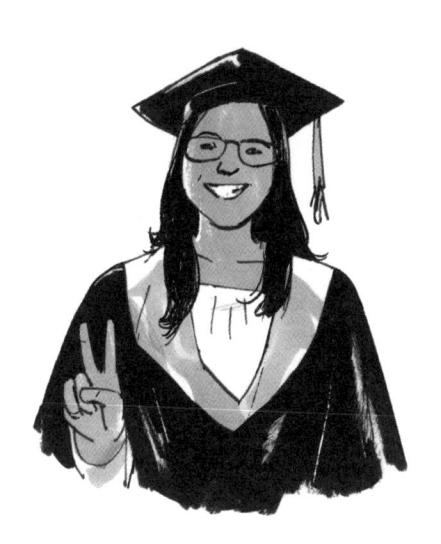

Across the park tremble-roars the
industrial hedge trimmer of the gardener,
who is cutting things back.

> A woman sits on a bench, a light breeze lifting
> the curls from her face, as she thoughtfully eats
> peanuts from a rustling, blue, foil bag.

A little girl feels the bark of a big, old tree
with her fingers. Occasionally, she places
her cheek against it and says what sound
like soothing things.

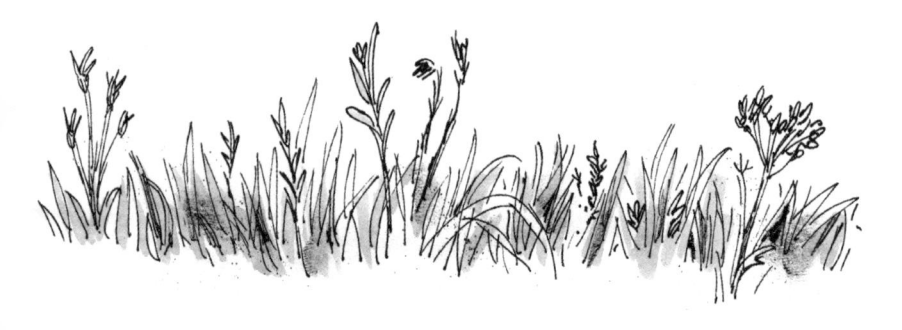

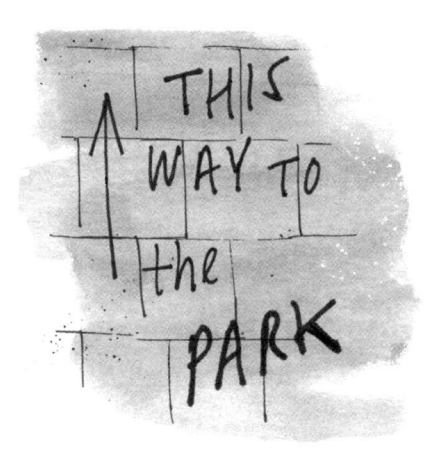

A silver-haired man in a black suit
sits under the old park bandstand
in the rain.

> In large, green, chalk letters
> on the pavement someone has
> stopped to write, 'This way to
> the park.'

IN A CAFÉ

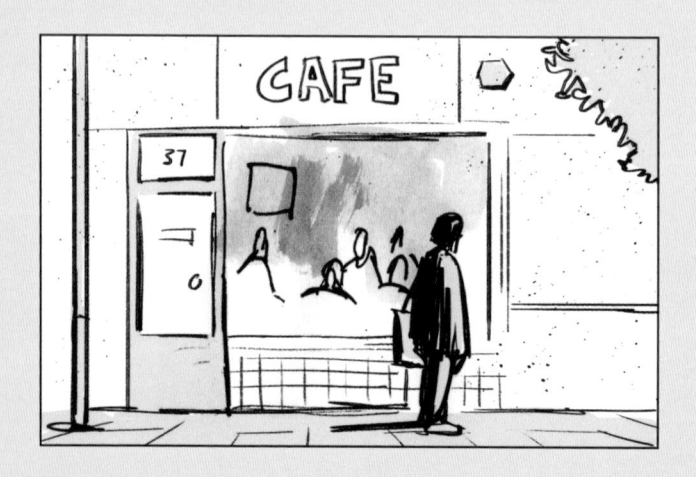

Cafés are more than places to eat or drink: they are offices, date venues, confessionals, somewhere to have a break while a baby finally sleeps.

I take in the layers as I approach. First, the outside – can I see my reflection in the glass? I look inside – is it full or empty? Are the tables close together? I zoom in. A baby sleeps in a pram. A pigeon has wandered in through the open door. I head in too, and choose a place to sit.

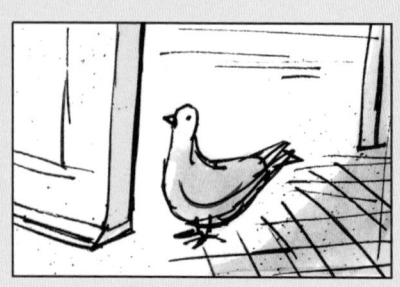

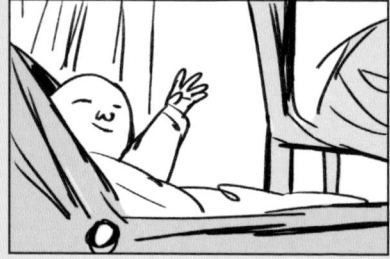

More intimate moments capture my attention: a person types on a laptop, their face lit by the screen. Someone puts a layer of ready-salted crisps inside their cheese sandwich. Someone buys a take-away coffee and runs out again. Their interaction is fleeting.

A regular wanders in. She leans on the counter and asks the owner about hisx kids. She isn't going anywhere for a while. Under it all is the sound of the drinks machine and the smell of coffee and toast.

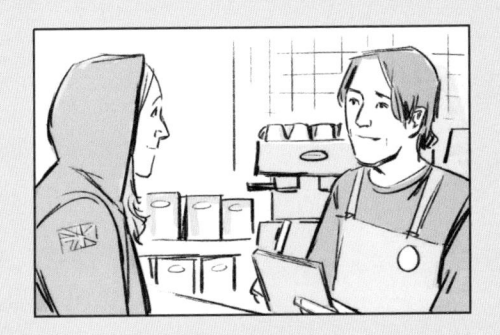

I zoom out. I notice the room again. It's a bit cold by the window. Wet trails from umbrellas cross the floor. I focus in. My notebook is open on the table in front of me. I turn a page in it. I write this.

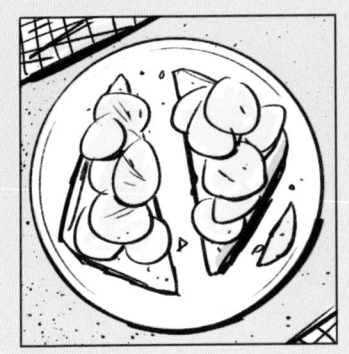

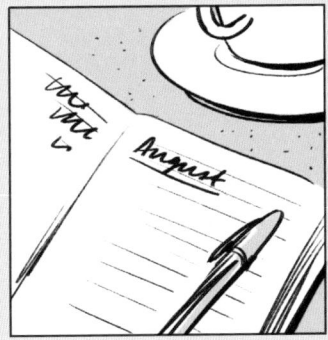

I am sitting in a café in Somerset House and my
table has a tree growing through it. I didn't notice
it when I chose to sit here, but now it is all I can
see. It is a tall tree – not a small, potted, table-top
decoration. I reach up to touch a leaf, half expecting
it to be plastic, but no, it is real. Around me, people
eat lunch, ignoring this outside-inside-tree.

Woman: Have you tried the cake?
Her friend: Yes. It's good. Really good.
But the slices are really big.
You'll want to share it.
Woman: No, I won't.

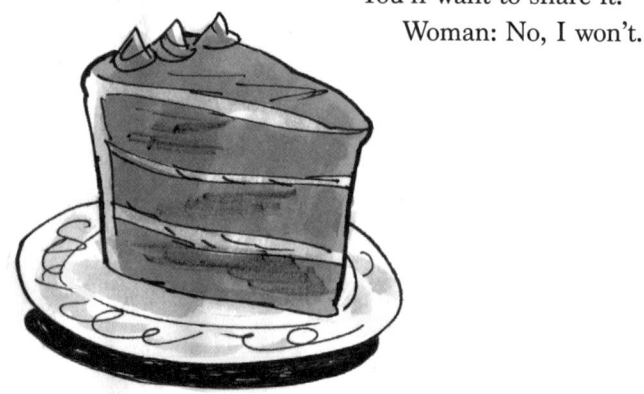

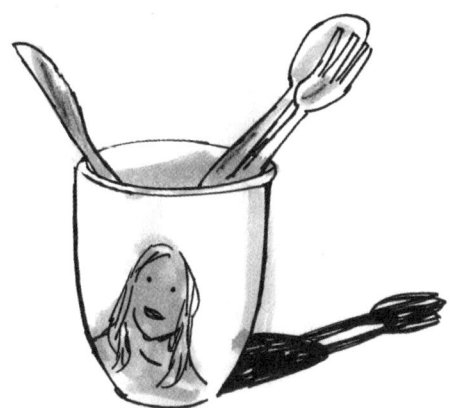

A man sits at a table beside me.
He talks about 'lived experiences'.
His hands make gestures in the air. I tune out of his
words, like moving a radio dial. I feel the hum of all
the voices surrounding me. I notice movements: a drink
being put down, a page being turned in a book. I notice
the dead wood of the floorboards, and think about the
bark and sap of the living tree growing through my
table. Cutlery leans drunkenly in a ceramic pot. The
glaze on the pot shows my reflection.

On a table near the counter, a man
dissects his eggs on toast with the air
of a disappointed surgeon.

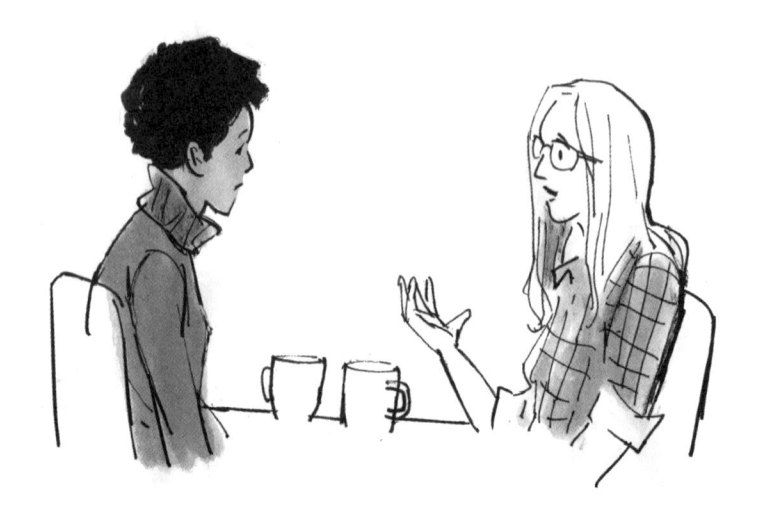

In a café in Brooklyn, New York, two women
talk at the table beside mine.
'How's your new apartment?'
'I love it. We're decorating. White walls and
black nail heads: monochromatic. But textural.
You know what I mean?'
'No...'

At a table for two in a café in Walthamstow,
I demarcate my space: a coffee and a small,
round cake provide a line, behind which I can
claim my area. My cake has four blueberries
on it, arranged like a three-petalled flower
– the centre fruit is the largest one. A lot of
thought has gone into this small snack.

Beside me, to the right, a woman types on a
laptop. She wears black. Her lips are painted
scarlet. Her pink socks say 'Surprise!' above the
line of her black boots. Suddenly she stops, takes
her hands from the keys and touches the opposite
tips of her fingers and thumbs together, as if
surrounding a grapefruit. Then she releases them,
to run rapid-fire again over the keys.

My friend: I love halloumi. Every
computer should have an 'order
halloumi' button.
Me: I'd never get any work done.

Waiter in a café: You're too late for breakfast
and too early for lunch.
Woman (to me): I'm sure there's a life lesson
here somewhere.

A woman working at the counter moves a Danish pastry with tongs from one part of the display to another, pauses, and then moves it back.

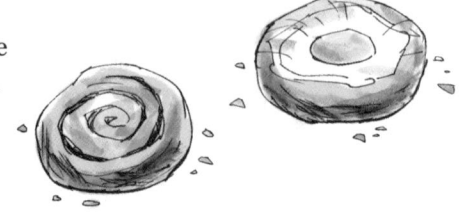

A woman sits, her laptop open. She's on a video call. In between the first and second knuckles of her forefinger and middle finger, she holds a pen. She makes a scissor action with her fingers so the pen rocks back and forth – the speed making an illusion, like wings growing out of her hand.

Woman returning to her friend at a table:
Sorry I was gone so long. It took me absolutely ages to get my Spanx back on.

I love the fact that every time the music
changes, the typing speed of the man nearest
me changes to match.

A black cat sleeps on the floor.
Shadows from the nearby chairs build
a house around her.

Man returning to his seat: Good God,
Margaret. That was, quite simply, the loudest
hand-dryer in the world.

A man talks to a friend. He emphasizes his points with his hands, positioning them like tall ships cutting through deep water.

A woman waits for a coffee in a coat that makes her look like a polar bear who has forgotten to put its head on.

As my toast arrives, the waitress asks: 'Miranda?' A woman opposite me also says, 'Yes.' We exchange a both-being-called-Miranda smile.

A barista places a man's coffee in front of him.
In the foam she has created a perfect swan, its
feathered wings spread wide. It is exquisite.
The man, not glancing up from his phone,
takes his first sip, and the swan is gone.

A little baby in a café does fabulous,
slow-mo, martial arts moves in her
high-chair to avoid the food her mum
is trying to feed her.

A woman working in a café rubs her pregnant
belly with her palm – a blue apron stretched over
the other person within her.

Sunlight falls across my table. The light picks out
many thin paper packets of sugar in their ceramic
bowl, casting a cactus-like shadow across the wood.

The place I'm in

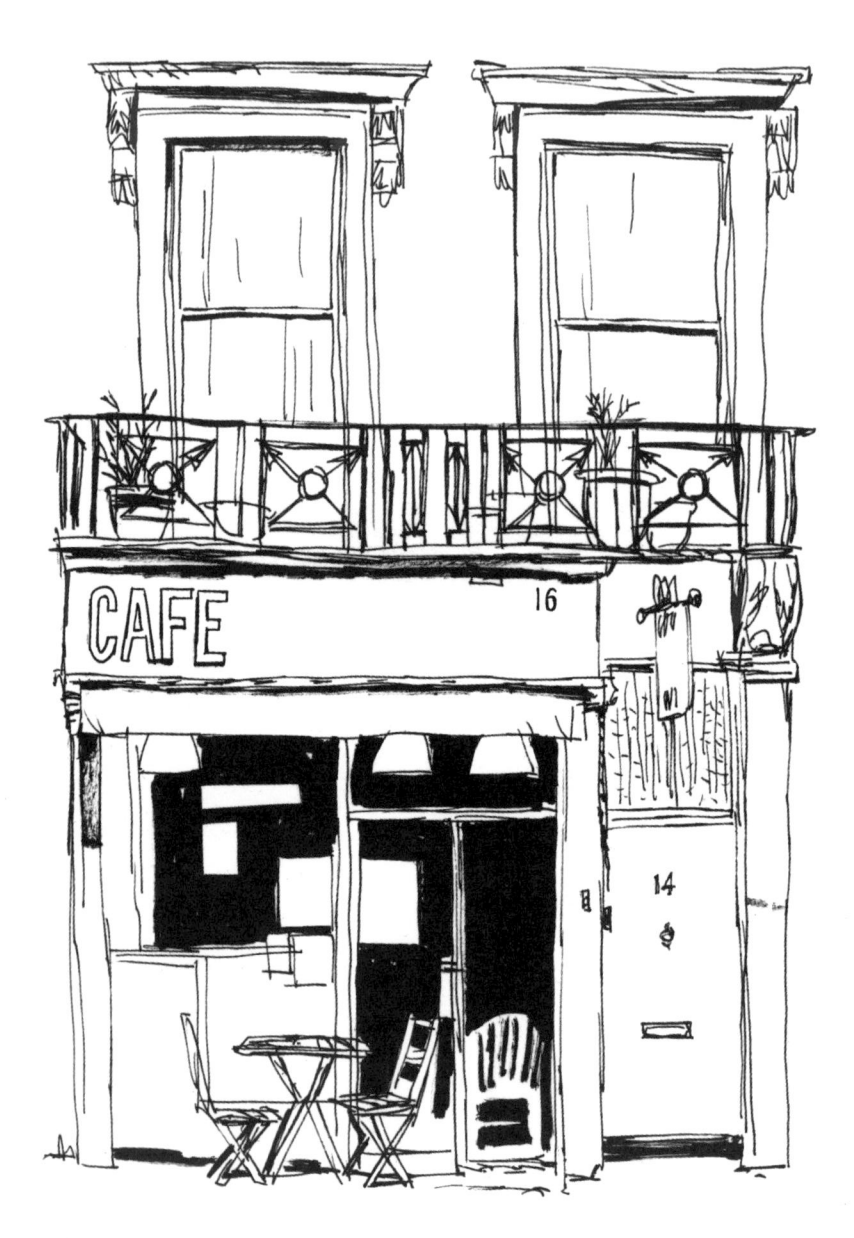

A toddler corrects a waitress's French.

A beautiful light appears in the eyes
of a woman sitting alone, as her friend
comes unexpectedly into the café and
notices her there.

A small boy is utterly entranced as his mum
flies a fork through the air with her hand,
and lands it on the table in front of him.

A woman takes a bite out of her sandwich. Around her plate are colour photographs of shells from which she has been sketching intricate illustrations in pencil.

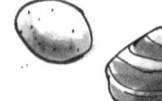

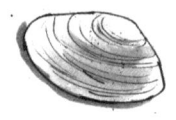

Man on a Zoom call in a café: Just before we finish up here, is that a gavel, John?'

A man working behind the counter places a heap of oranges by the juicer. He gives them a sympathetic nod in recognition of the onslaught to come.

I ask the waitress for a wheat-free wrap. She asks me why. I tell her I have an allergy. She says: Well, just so you know, the wheat ones are nicer.

A woman in a café in Birmingham talks to her
friend about something that is clearly annoying her,
from the intense way she is stirring her coffee.

A man with a wonderful white beard that juts
out from his chin like a snow shovel, peers at the
menu outside, his beard just shy of the glass.

I notice the yellow coat of a little boy sitting near me.
Me: Nice coat.
Little boy: Thank you. It means when night
comes I can hide as a star.

A woman walking to the loo runs her hands
over the pictures hanging in the hallway,
as if she is an air steward checking that the
overhead bag holders in the cabin are secure.

A woman outside the café seems to be
frantically waving at me and then I realize
that she is just cleaning the windows.

Man to his friend: Every day I buy the same
sandwich from the same café. Every day, the
same. It's only a cheese sandwich, you know.
But now it feels like coming home.

A red-haired woman reads an old paperback novel as if every word on the page is the most beautiful thing she's ever seen.

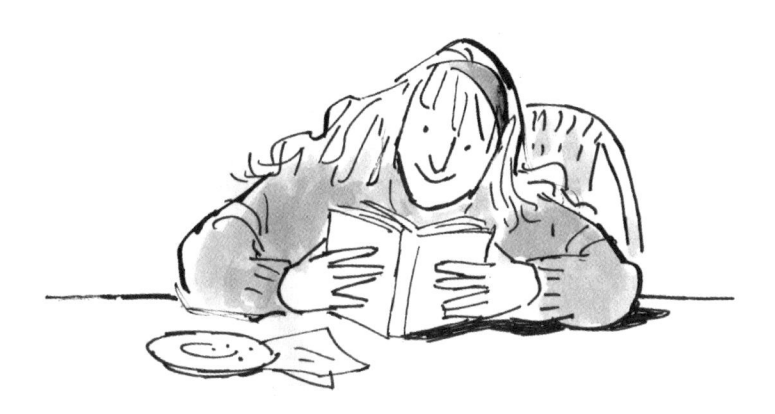

A teenager drinks a strawberry milkshake through a straw and then touches his forehead at his resulting cold-headache.

A woman at the counter stares down at the brownies on display as if eventually they will confess to something.

Man: I'd like the grilled cheese sandwich.
But I'd like to add potato. Is that weird?
Waiter: Whatever gets you through the day.

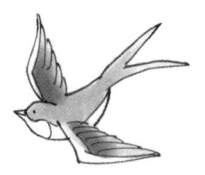

A little girl tries to coax a shy cat out from under
a table with a slightly squashed clementine.

A woman looks up from her laptop, sighs,
minutely adjusts the angle of a potted plant
on her table, and returns to work.

A woman in a café in Soho, who has ordered herself a salad, surreptitiously steals five of her friend's chips when he goes to the toilet.

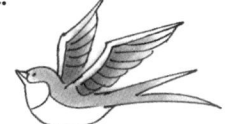

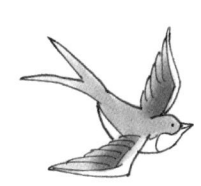

A woman makes coffee in a café in Brick Lane, many tattooed swallows in flight upon her freckled arms.

A woman sharing my table
talks to the man opposite her.
Woman: We have to be the adults in the
room, David. He will just have to accept that.
Man: That we are his parents.
Woman: That we are his parents.
Man: I mean we are.
Woman: Yes. Yes, we are.

ON THE STREET

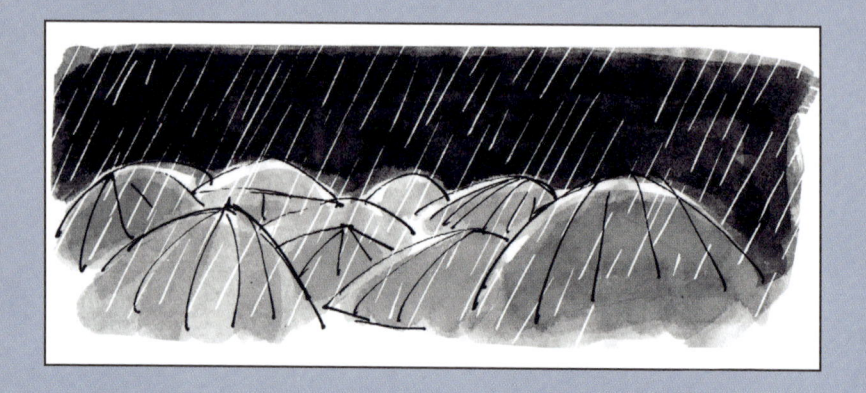

Outside things broaden. Boundaries stretch. Rain finds us walking the pavements as a bus passes, throwing a massive puddle over our best trousers – fresh on for an interview. The sun comes out. The sky is reflected again in the collected water, as its surface calms. The city provides a backdrop, even if we are rushing through it.

A man leans against a wall in the sun, drawing in charcoal the buildings opposite him across two pages of his sketchbook.

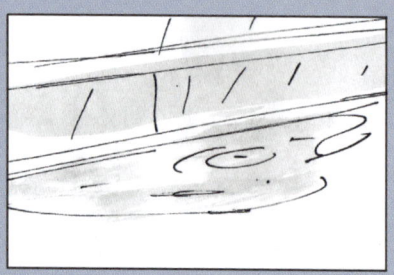

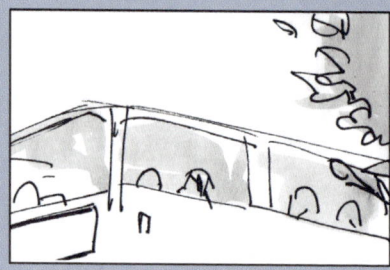

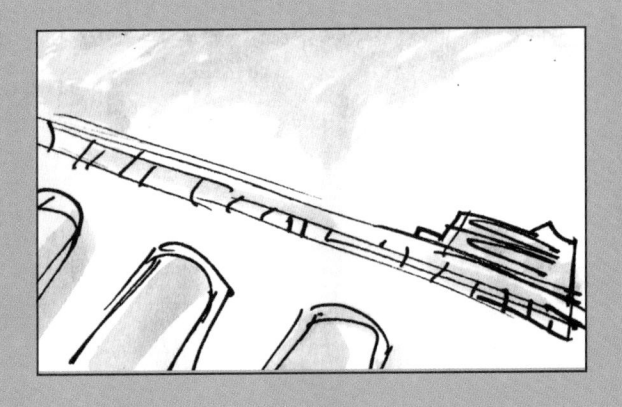

This is a liminal space. Sounds are different. They bounce hard off large buildings – streetscapes of masonry, brick and steel rather than café counters and pastry cabinets, rivers or blades of grass. A memory of my cat purring beside me on the sofa is tiny against the rush of things out here.

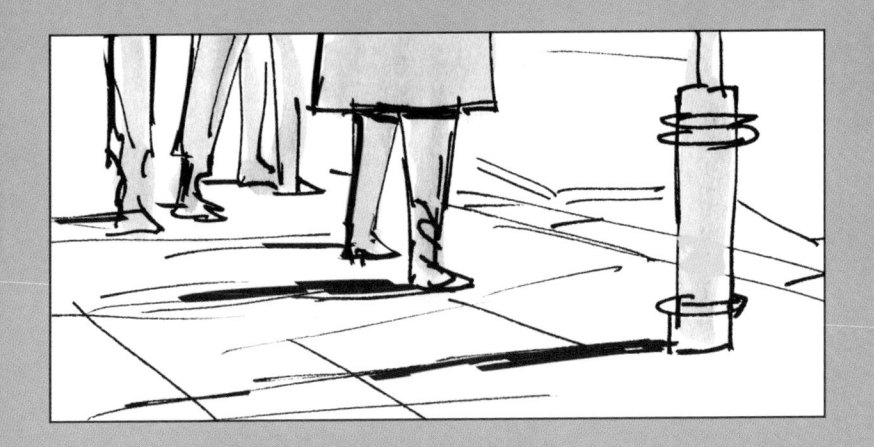

I stand in an alley looking up at the grey buildings stretching towards the sky. At the window of one room hangs a little row of pink bunting.

Outside a shop in Islington, something in the display makes many small lights fall across the grey pavement like electric snowflakes.

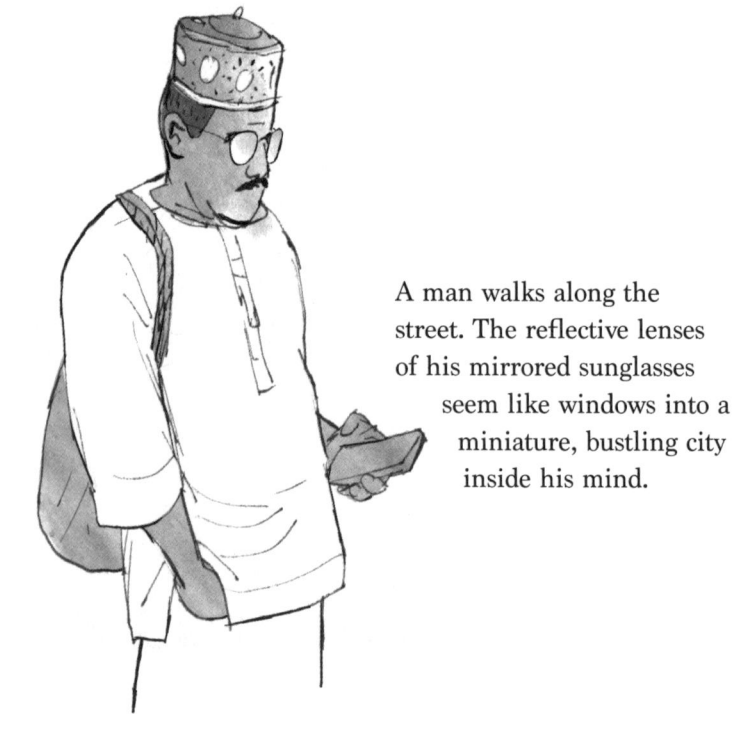

A man walks along the street. The reflective lenses of his mirrored sunglasses seem like windows into a miniature, bustling city inside his mind.

Two men unload green, plastic
crates of fizzy pop bottles from a van
into an Aladdin's cave of a space I never
knew existed behind a familiar shop.

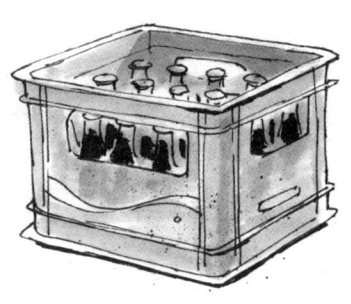

A woman in a shirt with a graph-paper pattern walks
a small, sand-coloured dog with a squashed, black
muzzle past the bench I'm on. She stops outside a
coffee stand and asks for a flat white. As she waits
for it, she starts to pace towards me and away again.
Her dog wants to smell my foot. It sniffs excitedly,
straining to touch its nose to my shoe, but it is on a
short lead and can't reach. I watch as the dog is pulled
away from me again. This repeats. I consider getting
up and presenting my foot to the dog to help out but
am not sure how this will look.

A man walks quickly. He wears triple denim and has an asymmetrical beard – longer on the right than the left. He talks into his phone: 'Alright mate, alright. I'm coming. I'm nearly there. I'm there.'

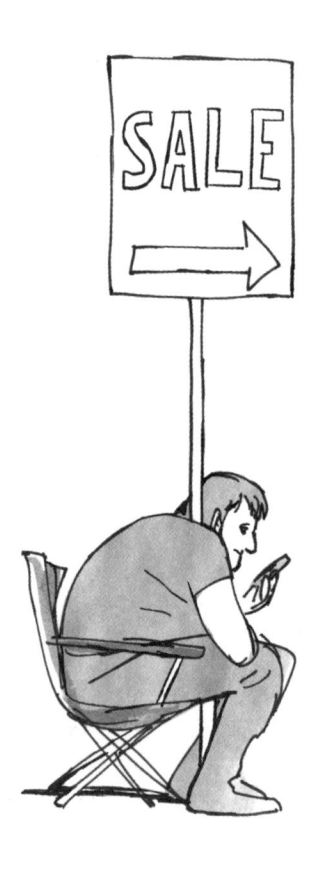

Another man comes out onto the street from a phone shop. He holds flyers. He inhales – the breath of one about to try and convince busy strangers to take a flyer today about phones. I know that breath. I have done my share of flyer-ing. He watches people walk. He offers the flyer to three passersby in a row. They do not acknowledge him.

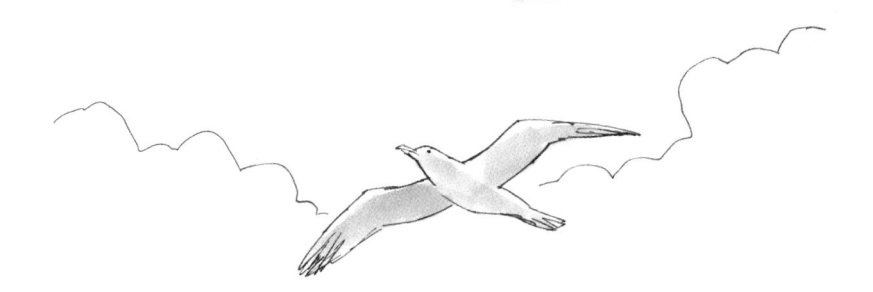

'Are You Lonesome Tonight?' plays somewhere.
A gull flies overhead.

I am concentrating on standing up in this wind. The hair of a woman crossing the road sticks straight out to the side and then whips in the other direction. The teal umbrellas outside a Caribbean restaurant judder and flare. Everything that can, moves. A man with a suitcase runs across the road. His face is flushed under his white hair. A long scar makes a crucifix of his left eyebrow. The wind tries to steal his suitcase, tearing his arm out to a 45-degree angle from his body. A woman tries to roll a cigarette and the contents scatter. A teacher with a gaggle of children counts them with a forefinger, and nods. None of them have blown away.

> A man walks past me with his arms crossed. His red and yellow rucksack is ancient and his trousers are frayed at the hems. In shoes too large for him, he places his feet as if trying to leave clear footprints on the pavement.

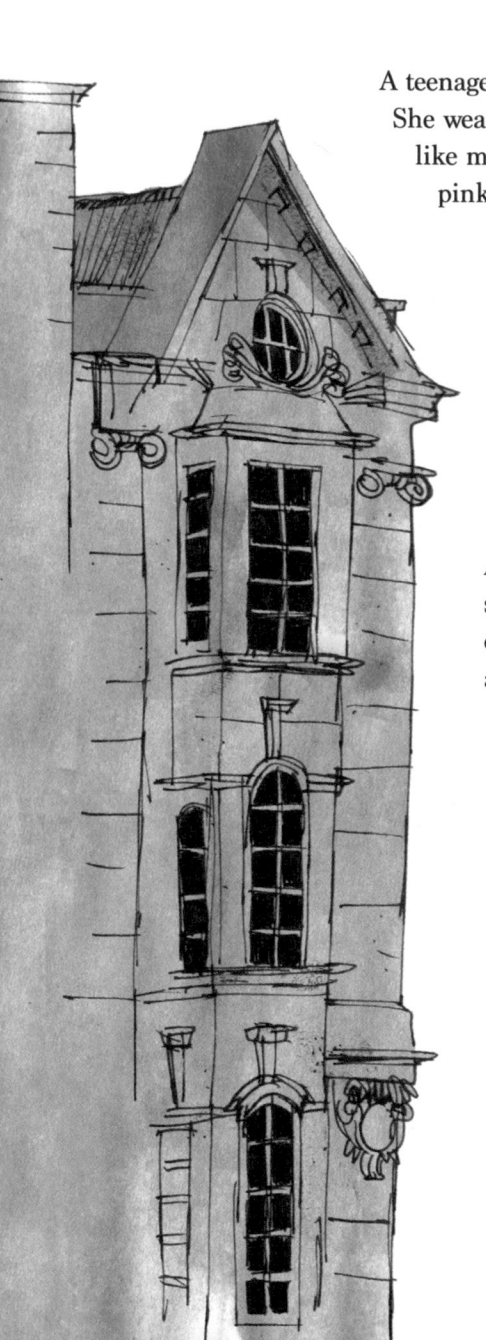

A teenager walks through Tottenham. She wears large, round, white earrings, like moons mid-orbit around the neon pink of her lipstick.

A street sweeper finishes smoking his cigarette, throws it on the floor, stubs it out, looks at it, nods and sweeps it up.

With absolute fascination, a little girl in a pram watches the rain-soaked pavement rush rapidly by below her yellow-wellied feet.

In the damp embrace of an old carpet is
a packet of unopened Turkish Delight.

Outside a scrapyard, a broken polystyrene
boat-cup floats across a muddy puddle to
an oil-slick rainbow on the other side.

A woman dressed in black on the
steps of a church suddenly stops
and takes a selfie at the front of a
funeral procession.

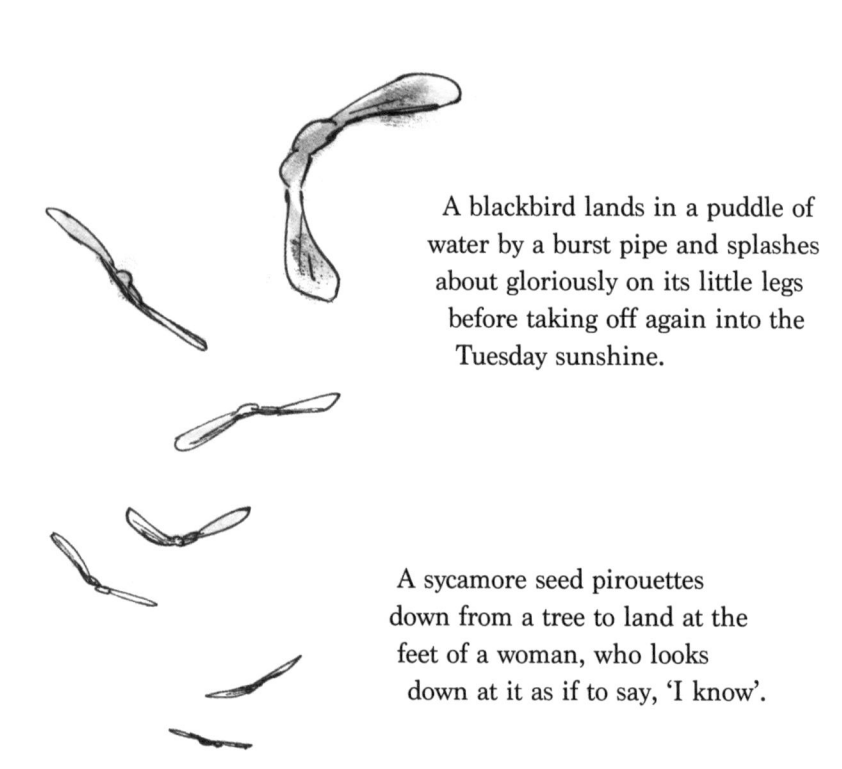

A blackbird lands in a puddle of water by a burst pipe and splashes about gloriously on its little legs before taking off again into the Tuesday sunshine.

A sycamore seed pirouettes down from a tree to land at the feet of a woman, who looks down at it as if to say, 'I know'.

I realize I am noticing types of walk today. A man walks past me, placing his feet very evenly. The whole of each sole touches the ground at once, not heel to toe or the reverse. I sit on the bench for a while longer in the sun.

A little boy insists on getting out of his pram to play the pavement with his blue-gloved fingers as if it's a piano.

Without realizing it, several people in Charing Cross instinctively walk in perfect time to a busker playing 'Stand By Me'.

From atop a building, stone women gaze down with pale grey eyes. Like brides in metal, pigeon-proof veils, they wait.

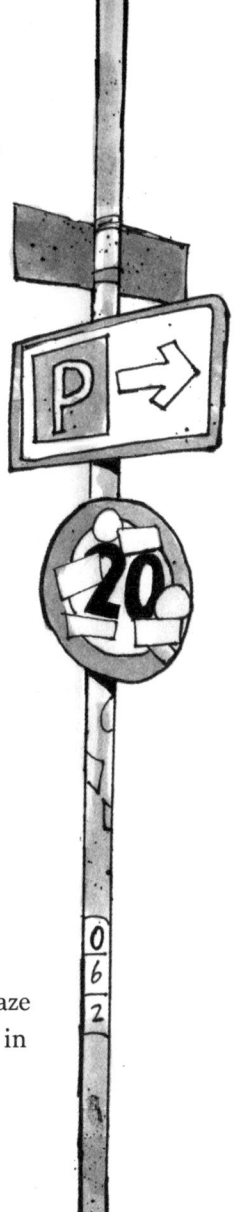

A man carries, with strange solemnity,
a surprisingly small square of pink
bubble wrap.

A very little girl stops on her scooter to stare
in wonder at the apples I am carrying inside
a rustling, clear, plastic bag.

A woman pushes a double pram. The
identical twin babies inside lean their
heads together until they are touching.

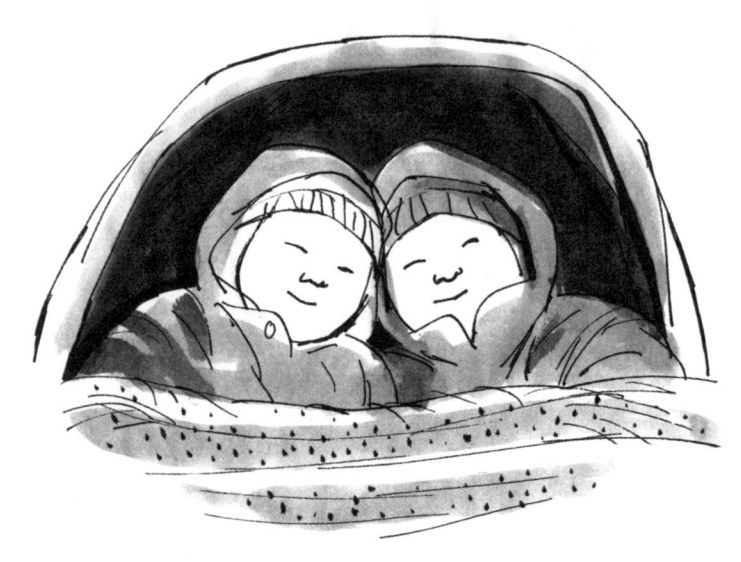

People watch a man cleaning upstairs windows on Wardour Street from the pavement with a very long pole, as if it is a wonderful circus act.

Woman looking at Tower Bridge: It's not just your average bridge, you know, this. I mean they've done something nice with it, haven't they?

A man is so distracted by a woman walking past him as he unlocks his front door that, when it opens, he falls into his flat.

Three fat, orange fish float lazily around their tank in a Chinese restaurant against a paper backdrop of some very hungry-looking sharks.

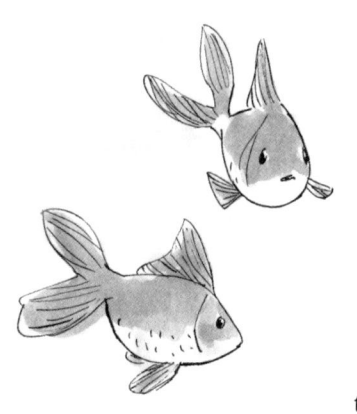

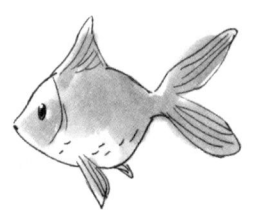

A lean man sprints through town, a broad smile on his chiselled face, long dreadlocks flying and yellow Day-Glo trainers on his swift feet.

Tourists in Baker Street gather excitedly in the falling rain to take photographs of the tall, grey statue of Sherlock Holmes.

A man paces up and down on a small patch of pavement staring into a lit window, a wooden rosary clasped tightly in his left hand.

A woman stands on one leg, talking to a friend while absentmindedly stretching the other leg up into a vertical split, bringing her foot almost to her ear.

At a window in Westbourne Park, a chandelier lights the room. One wall is covered in a large abstract painting in a metal frame. In front of the painting, a man wearing black does endless star jumps, a look of determination on his face.

Woman at a market stall: Those are labelled 'best avocados'.
Stall holder: Yes.
Woman: They're bruised.
Stall holder: See any better ones?

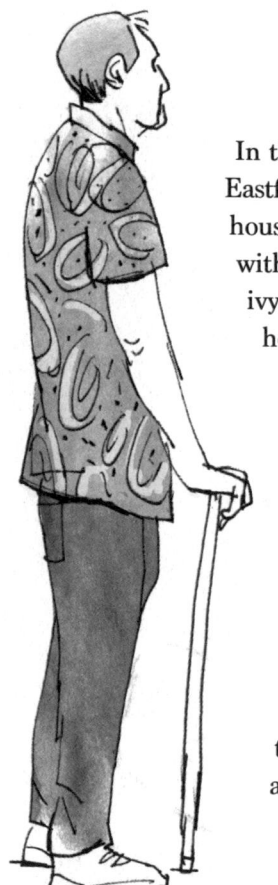

In the front garden of a house in Mitcham Eastfields, someone has built a second tiny house. It is about a metre high and perfect, with a beautifully tiled, pitched roof. Real ivy grows up the walls and, because the house is so small, the ivy leaves look strangely large against it.

A man in red jeans stands on a shop doorstep in Peckham, contemplating the pavement in front of him, as if it is a very long way down.

A man in a white, knitted jumper, his eyes serenely closed, dances with a folded-up umbrella to the Motown music coming from a nearby market stall.

Several pine cones play caught-by-the-wind kiss-chase, with an empty, purple packet of Cadbury's Mini Rolls.

A group of security guards stand outside an office block on a break, meticulously working out which one of them has the longest arms.

A man walks across Waterloo Bridge, hugging an old rolled-up newspaper to his chest and muttering soothingly to it, 'It's ok, it's ok.'.

A woman minding a flower stall is on a loop of jolting awake, checking the flowers, adjusting her glasses and falling asleep again.

A mum at traffic lights smiles as her little boy pushes the button with the tiny paw of his soft-toy dog.

A man walks without shoes along Nørre Voldgade in Copenhagen, with his blonde hair in a bun and the dust of the streets on his feet.

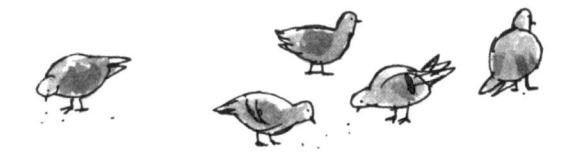

A woman walks down the street in a tie-dyed shirt. Her rolled-up sleeves reveal arms covered with tattoos of faces whose eyes remain open as she rubs hers with thumb and forefinger.

A little boy leans out of a window to wave at a woman's dog.
Woman: Don't make him bark.
Boy: Don't speak back, dog, but how're you?

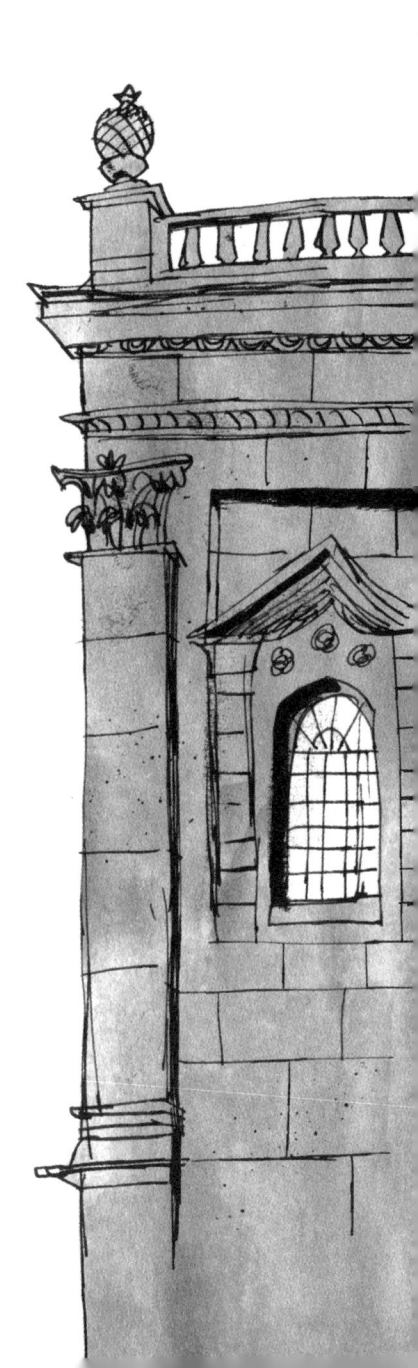

POPPING IN

When I pop in somewhere, I notice the things I need to – a sign above an aisle, the entrance to an exhibit, the till. I often head in with one purpose and find that something else grabs my attention. Popping in has a casual nature to it, like a physical form of mind-wandering.

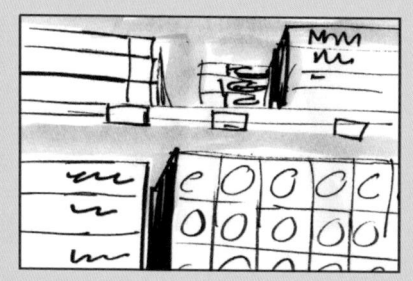

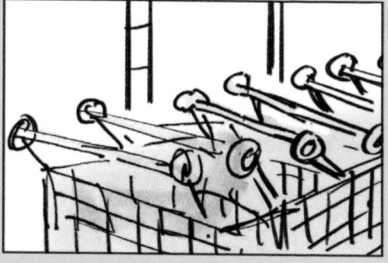

In shops people scan shelves, lugging around over-filled baskets – they only came in for 'a few bits', but you know what it's like. They bump into a neighbour in the cheese aisle and pause to catch up. Their dog whines for them outside.

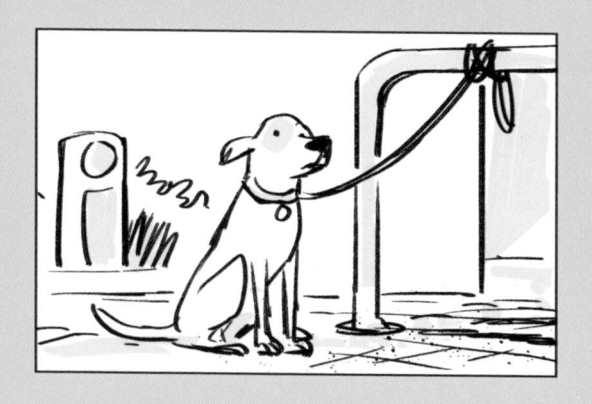

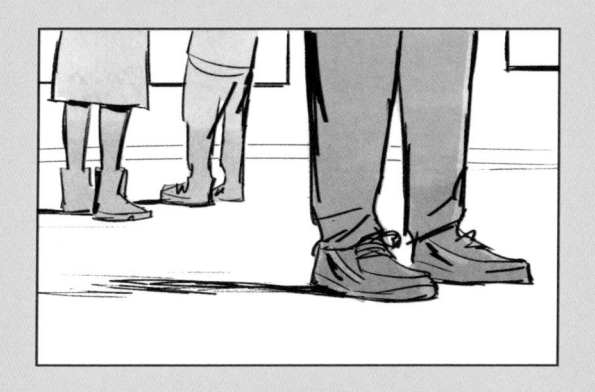

When you find folk focused on specific tasks, you sometimes have a little window into their lives – from what's in their trolley to the items they put back or impulsively throw in.

The hush of a museum or a library means I observe different things – sound especially: the squeak of trainers on a polished floor, muted conversation, the delighted giggle of a baby.

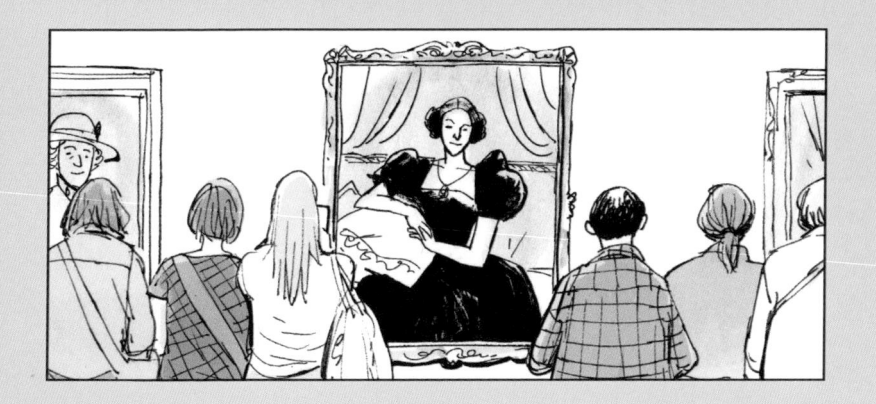

In the Horniman Museum in south London, a large taxidermy walrus is stuck to a pretend iceberg. It has apparently been on display for more than a century. Its dark toes are splayed, long tusks emerge from its dead mouth to curve gently towards its chest and where once there was fur there is now mostly leathery brown skin.

Woman to her little boy: Ooh, look at those teeth. Shall we take a photo of you by the walrus for Daddy?

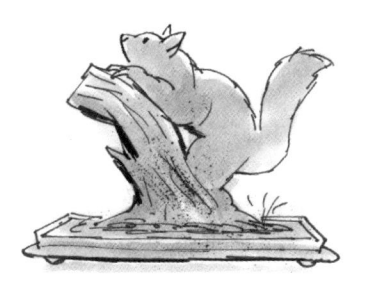

A man walks past. He is tall and veins stand out on his forearms. He uses a white stick to feel his way through the museum. As he passes the things in tall, glass cases, the woman he is with tells him what they are: Possum. Hoary Tree-Porcupine. Murex Scolopax. Sea Mat. Spotted Globe Fish. Cockroach.

> Woman in a museum in Oxford (opening part of an interactive display about English rural life): Oh no. I've found the myxomatosis drawer.

> Little boy looking into the royal railway carriage at the Shildon Railway Museum in County Durham: Posh.

In an Asda in Lewisham, a man on a
mobility scooter is dressed for fishing; he
wears a broad-brimmed khaki hat with a
flap to cover the back of his neck and a
strap with a toggle under his chin. He wears
ripstop combat trousers and a waterproof
camo jacket with a chest pocket. The jacket
is open and inside is a fishing vest with lots
of smaller pockets. The fish in this Asda are
already caught. As far as I know.

Two women in the alcohol aisle are pretending it is
their personal bar and are ordering drinks from each
other. They walk across the lino as they choose,
flip-flops flapping against their heels.
Woman 1: What'll you have?
Woman 2: A daiquiri. And a decaf espresso martini. You?
Woman 1: An advocaat. And a double Crème de Menthe.
Do you do snacks?

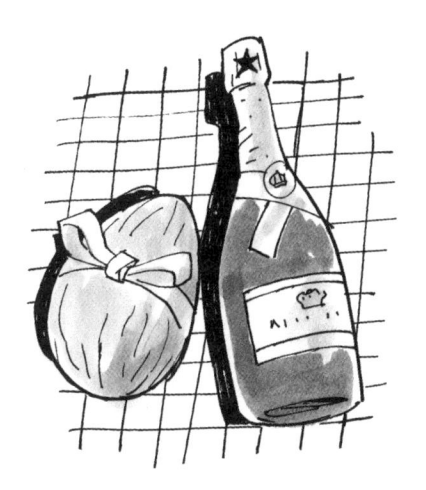

A dad turns around to see his toddler carefully placing two items into the trolley: a chocolate egg and a bottle of pink champagne.

In a supermarket in South London, a man with a peaceful face waltzes to in-store music. His dancing partner is a small loaf of ginger cake.

Man behind the till: That's £64.
Woman: Gosh.
Man: I'm sorry.
Woman: It's not your fault.

A mum in Foyles bookshop, holding her tiny
baby in a papoose, blows air across his forehead
in order to keep him calm while she reads.

Woman near the café in an art
gallery: Oh, thank goodness!
Man: What's that?
Woman: I can smell tea.

A shop assistant, entirely dressed as
an enormous silver Christmas cracker,
absentmindedly arranges nappies on a shelf.

84 ● The place I'm in

I look through the photos I took at the
Museum of Childhood (now the Young V&A)
in Bethnal Green. In one, of a dolls' house, a
woman is reflected in the glass cabinet, placed
perfectly into one of the rooms. She is bent
at the waist and only just fits, like Alice in
Wonderland after a bite of cake.

> Every time a mum in the museum loo starts
> to tell her little boy off, he puts his hands
> under the hand-drier so he can't hear her.

I pass the fisherman on his mobility scooter
again. He is waving his hand at the energy
drinks dismissively. He slows to a stop by
the tinned fish and stares it down.

A member of staff at the V&A gives me directions. She goes into such loving detail in her reply, saying things like, 'When you get to the spot where the sunlight falls in a great slant across the delicate ironwork, turn left,' and it makes my heart soar.

The lift opens. There is no room to get in. For the time that the doors remain open, I am presented with a fantastic freeze-frame of humanity.

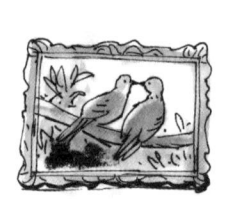

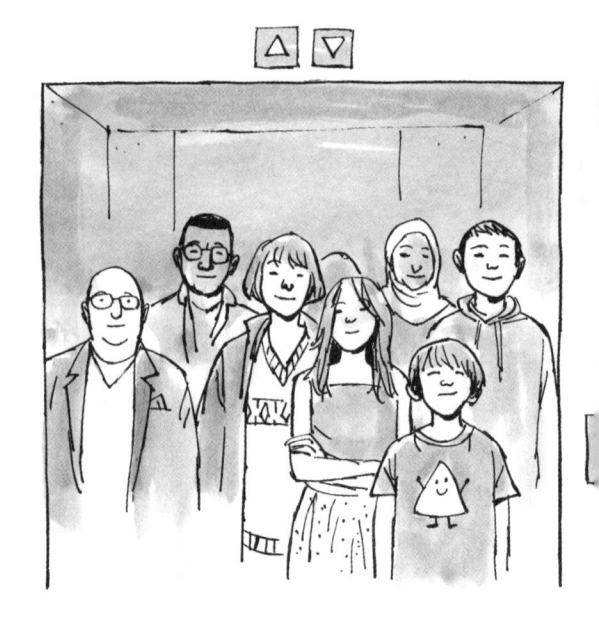

Two men are sitting together in a display bath in John Lewis and laughing at the fact they are there.

A woman working behind the front desk does her best imitation of looking happy, as a late visitor is let in just before closing time.

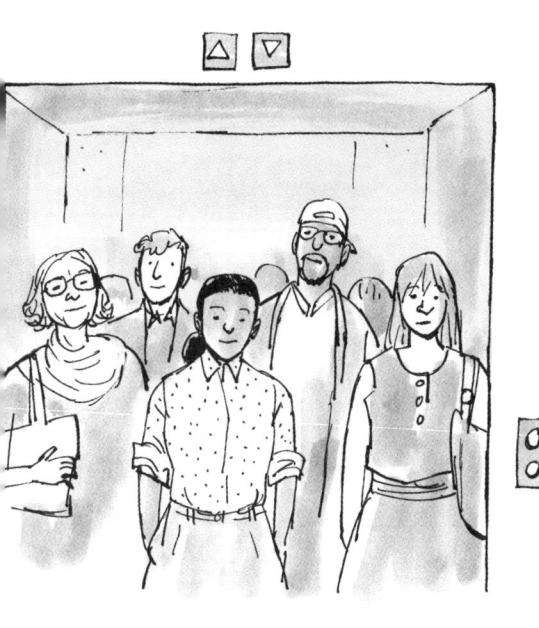

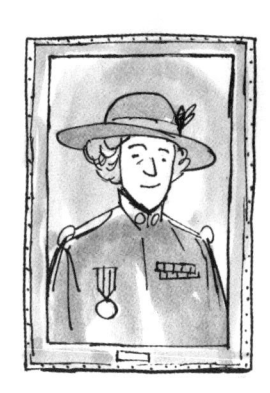

Popping in

A man holds a museum door open for a woman to come through.
Woman: Thank you. One hundred to come.
Man: Sorry?
Immediately, the many schoolchildren she is responsible for begin to come through the door behind her.
Man (exhaling and settling in for the long haul): Ah.

Outside, a large, oily, rainbow-surfaced bubble floats slowly past a security guard.

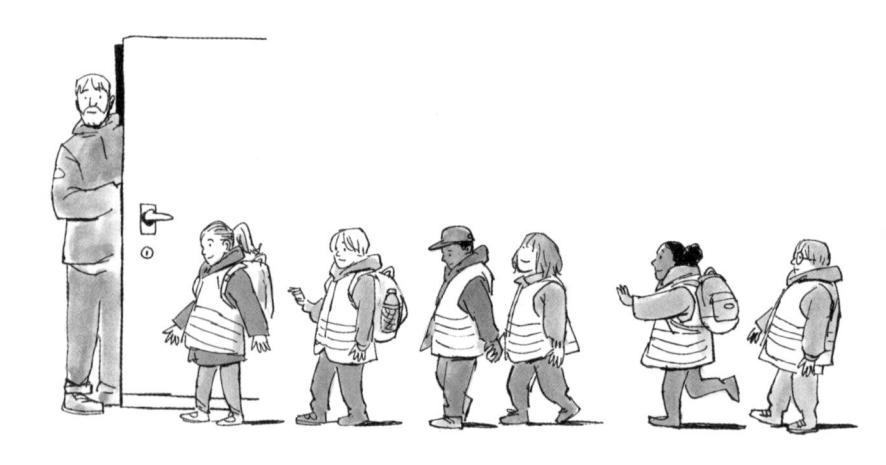

A bored little boy in the stationery section in a shop in Hackney turns a tube of wrapping paper into a megaphone, a telescope, a walking stick, a ray gun and a flute.

A man and a woman discuss politics while picking out plantains for their dinner with practised ease.

A man jogging through the city finds it impossible to ignore a lovely, stripy jumper in a shop window, and jogs in to try it on.

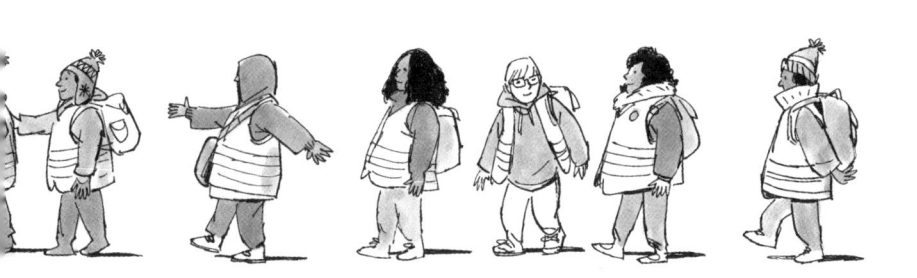

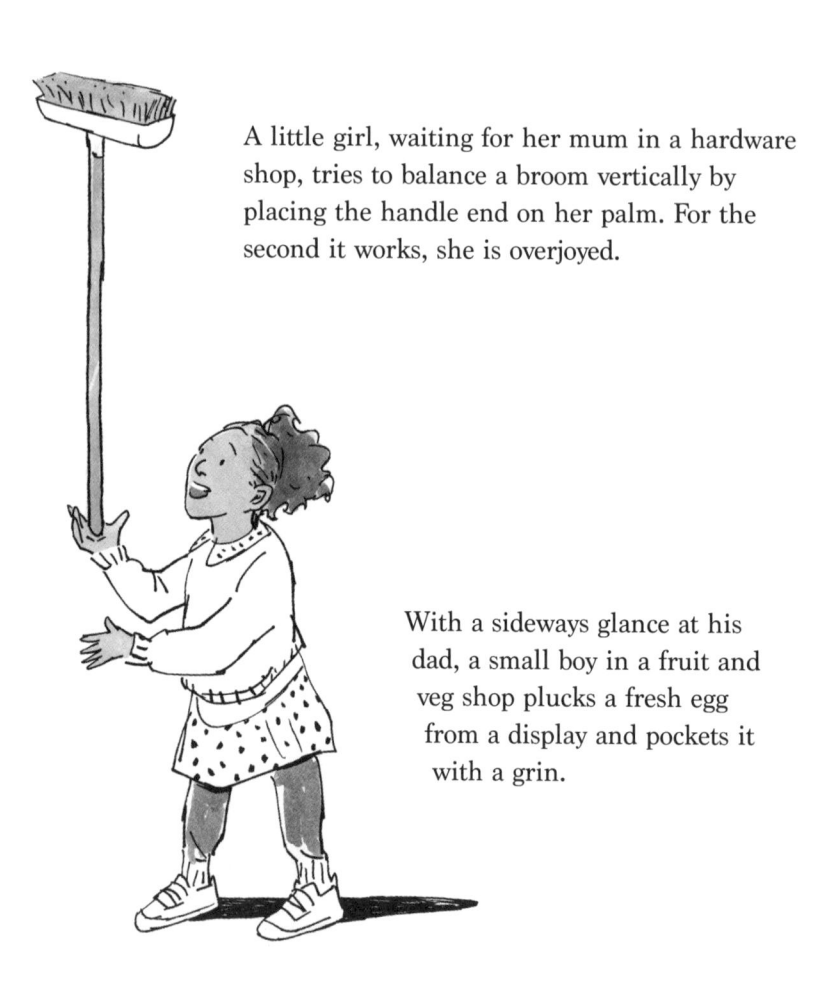

A little girl, waiting for her mum in a hardware shop, tries to balance a broom vertically by placing the handle end on her palm. For the second it works, she is overjoyed.

With a sideways glance at his dad, a small boy in a fruit and veg shop plucks a fresh egg from a display and pockets it with a grin.

Teenager walking past a display of doughnuts in a bakery (to his friend): Note that.

A man sits on the floor of a bookshop absorbing
the details of a graphic novel as if they're water
and he is in great need of a drink.

                                         A white-haired woman on a ladder
in a gift shop strikes fabulous,
contemporary-dance-type poses as
she puts new batteries into a clock
on the wall.

A man in a kebab shop prepares an order
for take-away. He finishes by rolling the
kebab in silver foil with a flourish, and
nodding to his waiting driver – it's ready.

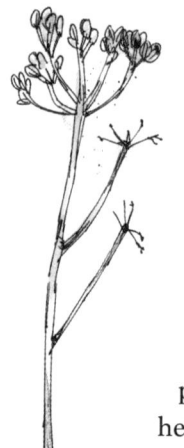

During the moments I spend choosing a plant at my local garden centre, a teeny, tiny spider begins to spin a web between me and a sunflower.

In an Italian deli, a little girl behind her dad pulls dramatically on imaginary reins to bring her pretend horse to a sharp stop by the cheese.

Man in a newsagent: This water is labelled 'gluten-free'.
Till guy: Yes.
Man: It's water.
Till guy: It's gluten-free water.

A woman in a black burka stands in a fabric shop on Berwick Street stroking a piece of shiny, silver, sequin-covered cloth.

A man in a shop wears red, silver and black cowboy boots, a furry orange coat and a purple velvet hat. I tell him that his look is great. He nods and says, 'Glad you dig it.'

A sturdy-looking dog wearing army camouflage waits outside a shop in Camden. Between his teeth he is holding a large, orange, rubber chicken.

A woman outside stops in her tracks on noticing the window display, as she exclaims excitedly to herself, 'Ooh, buckets!'

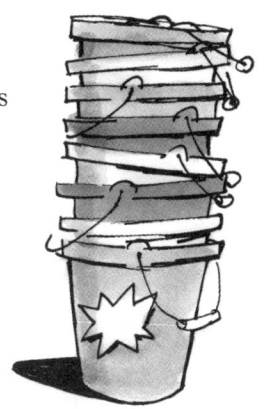

A cab driver leaps from his taxi into a
nearby coffee shop, howling with shock at
the pouring rain that pelts him on the way.

                    A man working in a chip shop serves chips in
                    time with the dance music playing on the radio
                    and it is a surprisingly pleasing thing to watch.

A person buying cake in a cake shop
(with a very irritated tone): You
mean you can't write anything on it?
The woman working there silently
passes them a pen.

                    Assistant in a shop: Did you want this hat, then?
                    Older woman: No, love, the nights are drawing
                    in, I'm tired, and anyway, it's hideous.

A homeless man sits outside a shop in Southend. His dog sleeps beside him in the sun. The man finishes the hard sudoku in the *Metro*. He glances up with satisfaction, and we exchange a grin.

Woman in the NEMO Museum in Amsterdam (reading the information tags on a display from the 1700s): Lady's companion.
She locates the corresponding item.
It is a sewing kit.
Woman: Ah, disappointing.

A woman in a wheelchair is pushed to sit beside the bench I'm on in the Horniman Museum. Her companion walks over to look at the walrus. I smile at the woman. She smiles back, lines shooting across her cheeks. She points to the case beside us. She reads the names: Sloth. Pangolin. Tree-frog. We nod at each other.

IN THE COUNTRYSIDE

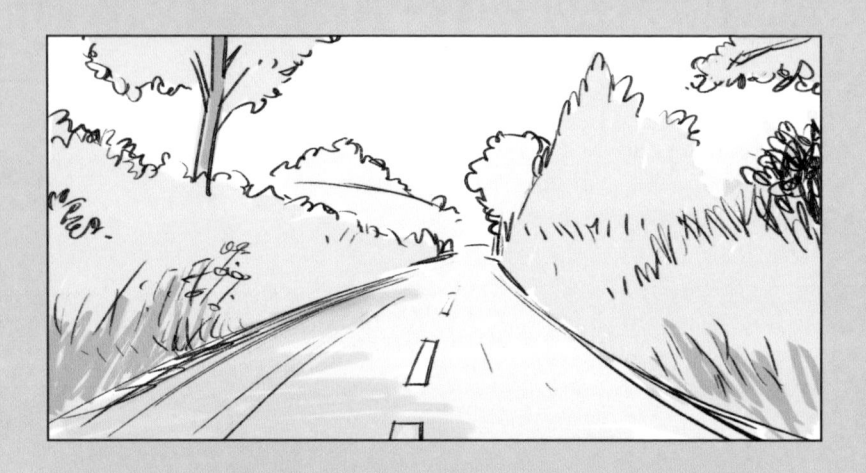

Trying to describe the countryside makes me aware of the gaps in my knowledge. With fewer people and buildings to notice and fewer conversations to eavesdrop on, I'm left looking up names of trees, shrubs, clouds or animals.

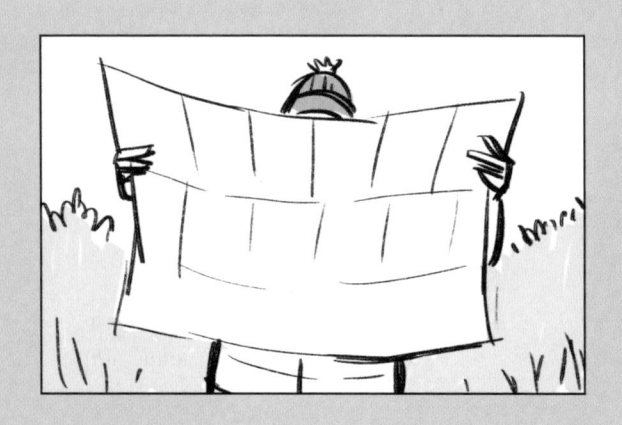

Street signs no longer demarcate the space. Instead, I use my phone to find the names of rivers and woodland.

If there's no reception, I must plan where I'm going beforehand or carry a paper map. This changes the way I understand the world around me. I'm left with only the words I already have to describe a mushroom or a particular kind of lichen. Perhaps this makes me more connected to the place I'm in. Not being able to refer to a Dryad's Saddle doesn't stop me appreciating the way a large mushroom's broad cap looks like a hand-thrown, shallow bowl, its edges undulating. I can't post these observations online instantly, and get real-time responses. Instead, the words must wait inside my notebook.

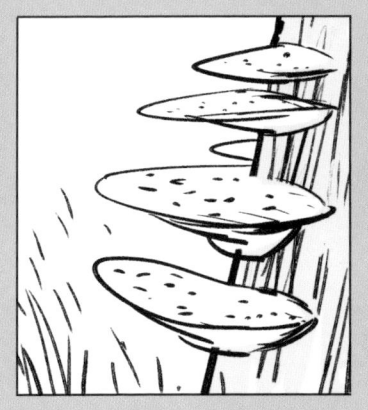

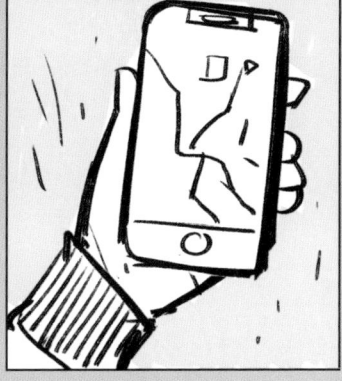

As I see further and the view becomes less crowded, the brushstrokes of my noticings become broader and simpler. I exhale, and with it my writing changes a little, too.

Woman on a bus in Hackney (staring at the traffic): I want to go to the countryside. Stand on a hill. Look out at the world. And breathe.

Rain falls against this train, the sound like grains of rice poured into a bucket. A veil of grey covers the fields beyond the window.

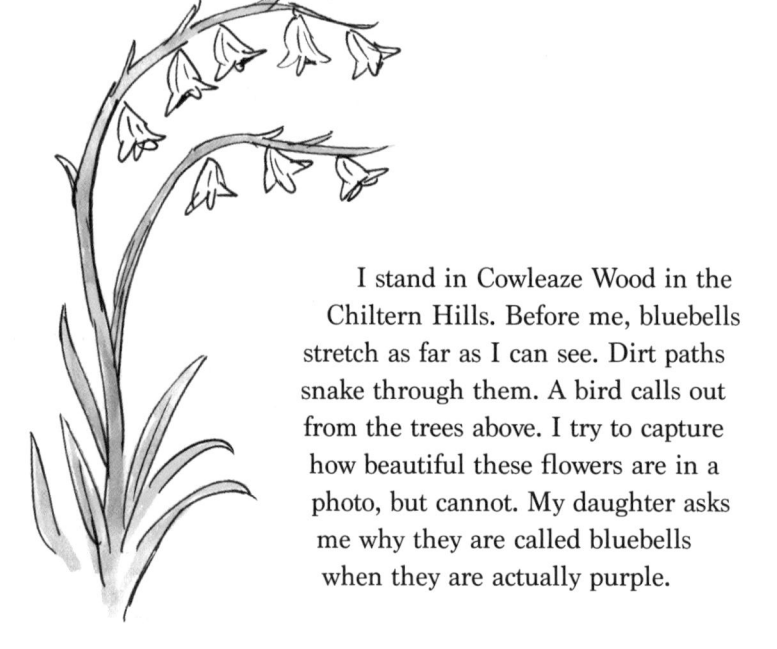

I stand in Cowleaze Wood in the Chiltern Hills. Before me, bluebells stretch as far as I can see. Dirt paths snake through them. A bird calls out from the trees above. I try to capture how beautiful these flowers are in a photo, but cannot. My daughter asks me why they are called bluebells when they are actually purple.

Mist hangs over Glastonbury as I begin my walk up the Tor.

Over a lake in the Catskill Mountains in New York State, there are so many stars. The late-summer chill reaches through my jumper. I can hear a mosquito by my right ear – that irritating squeal-whine. Before me, Cooper Lake is black and almost indistinguishable from the land – an oil spill on fresh tarmac.

A man sits on a fallen tree near Kingston in New York State. He is crocheting something orange. The pointy tip of his long, brown beard keeps trying to become part of what he is making.

A feeding trough in a field in
Oxfordshire is painted red. The colour,
combined with the shape of its openings,
reminds me of London's buses.

Little boy near Denby Dale, West Yorkshire,
looking at a large black and white dog: Oh
dear, has anyone told him he's cow colours?

A bespectacled man alone on a bench near
Cambridge keeps finding himself utterly
overwhelmed by sudden, silly giggles.

A woman walks through the woods. A bright, copper, splatter-pattern creeps up the back of her black leggings. Either that or she is an alien who has been here for too long and her costume is wearing thin.

Mushrooms emerge from tree trunks sideways, as if sidling into place surreptitiously.

Gulls flock around a hole in the ice of a frozen-over river somewhere on the way to South Shields, Tyne and Wear, as the morning sun makes diamonds of the frost.

Little girl in the woods: He's talking!
That dog is talking to us, Mummy!
Her mum: He is? What's he saying?
Little girl: Woof, woof.

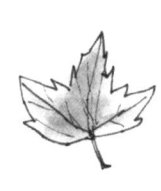

A woman walks through puddles in her wellies.
The puddle bottoms are full of leaves – the water's
surface reflecting back the trees they fell from.

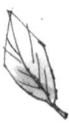

A woman stops outside the postbox to count
the number of Christmas cards in her hand,
before smiling to herself and posting them.

A very small baby in a pram is entirely swaddled
in purple fleece, apart from her sleeping face and
one tiny, orange, stripy-socked foot.

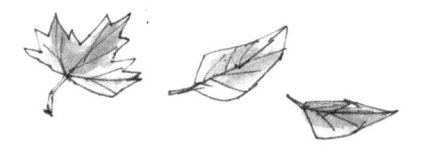

A grey-haired woman walks through the rain,
her red leather-gloved hands clasped behind her
back, her eyes bright with a detective-like gleam.

As the evening gets chillier, the windows of
a village pub mist up in patches, making it
look like it's full of rotund, ghostly patrons.

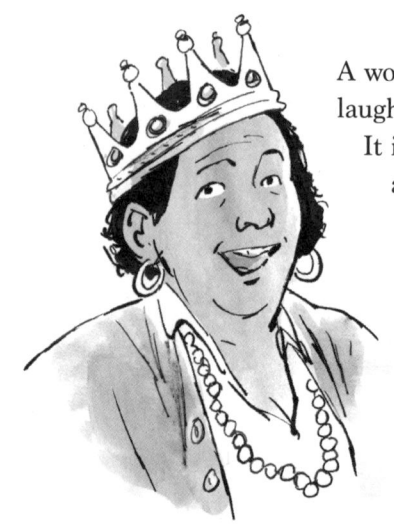

A woman outside the pub entrance laughs. She wears a plastic crown. It is gently askew. She doesn't appear to mind.

A grape-shaped man walks in the woods. His dark blue jumper is snug around his middle, his neck is hugged by a bright purple scarf and white shoes swamp his surprisingly small feet. His companion is an elderly, brown dog.

Woman in the woods (to her dog): Oh Gwilym, we've been through this: if you don't release the ball from those considerable jaws, I cannot throw it for you.

Lichen blooms on a fallen oak in the woods. At the toppled tree's highest point, a crow stands, looking down at another crow beneath it, with perhaps the bird equivalent of contempt.

I stand beside the Mallyan Spout waterfall in Goathland, North Yorkshire. The water pours down the rock, forming spindles as if it has suddenly frozen into icicles on this warm day.

By the West Beck river in the Yorkshire Wolds, a tree trunk lies. Its sides are covered in pennies hammered into the soft wood. The resulting texture is otherworldly – a scaly, bark-coated, crocodile-thing.

Two men sit silently together on chairs in a side
street in Nyons in the south of France. Above
them, a sign tells me that a house is for sale. As
I always do, whether the sign is far from where I
live or simply on another house on my own street,
I move there in my mind for a few moments,
leaving my own home behind.

> Everyone else is inside on this August day in
> Mirabel-aux-Baronnies, near Avignon, France.
> The sun presses against my back as I walk
> to the supermarket. Wooden shutters – the
> houses' eyelids – are closed against the heat.
> Dry leaves, picked up by a brief gust of wind,
> gather around my sandalled feet.

As I face the Cascade d'Aubres in the
south of France, light comes through the
foliage in little sparks and bursts. A small
boy sits on the stones eating a peach.
Spray from the waterfall flattens his hair.
The air is full of the roar of falling water.

Water flows along a creek in Woodstock, Oxfordshire. As light falls on the forest floor, the leaves in its path make grey lace of the resulting shadows.

A little girl climbs the stones of Hadleigh Castle in Essex to place her soft-toy rabbit at a window. Presumably this gives the rabbit an excellent view across the fields that dip down towards the Thames Estuary.

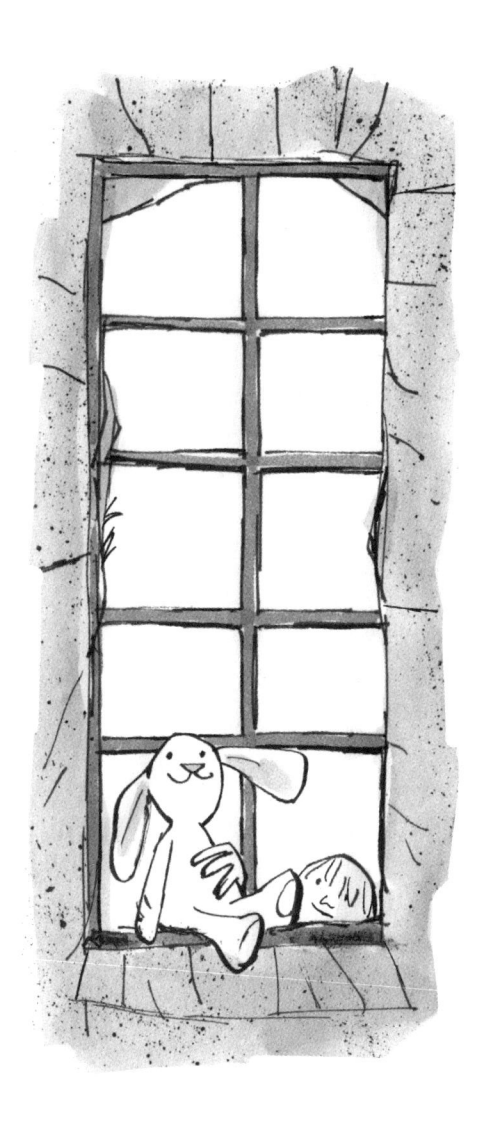

A man carries his small, brown dog up the final three steps to a ruined abbey. The dog rests across the man's shoulders like a stole, its expression regal. The sky peers with her brilliant, blue face through the great, arched windows of the abbey remains.

Ivy grows through a wooden church fence in that way it has of determinedly pushing beyond its borders. Some of its leaves are green, while others are brown and stiffened. Birds sing from trees in the graveyard. A woman tells her friend she is so excited about something that's going to happen.

At a craft fair in Devon, a phone rings. A woman turns her head towards it. Attached to her jumper, a ceramic hedgehog brooch looks in the opposite direction.

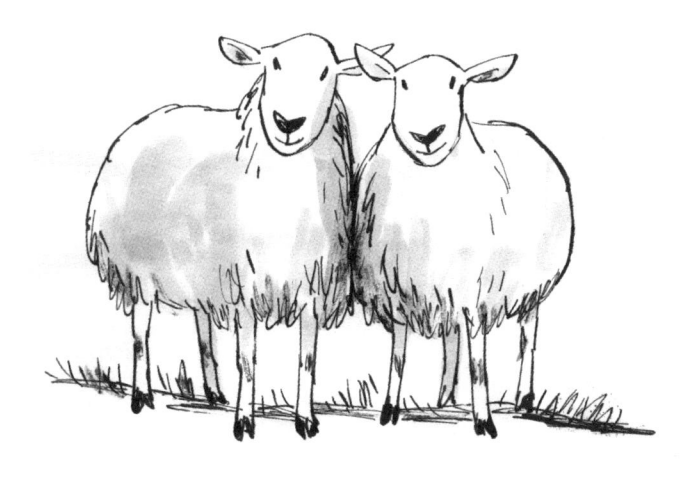

Sheep graze in a field near Buckingham. Two of them stand beside each other, woolly flanks touching.

Selected stones have been balanced into bottom-heavy towers upon Lindisfarne's brilliantly blustery shore.

Little boy on Holy Island, Northumberland, looking towards the causeway: I hope the sea doesn't come in and eat our car.
His dad: Me too, son. Me too.

In the countryside

Selsley Common in Stroud brings me words
as I stand in the middle of it: far, wide, large,
stretching. People walk across the grass at such a
distance they could be in my imagination. The sky
above seems to curve at the edges. I feel as though
I am in a gift shop globe that someone will turn
over and back up, as snow begins to fall.

All along the banks of Durham's
River Wear, the tall trees are trading
in their summer clothes of green for
the reds and golds of winter.

In the moonlight, I manage to make out the
face of a girl on her houseboat, and she flashes
me a smile through the deepening dark.

A grey squirrel forages on the forest floor – as his
nose goes down, his tail springs up magnificently.

On a country road, a man uses a remote control
to open his front gate as he approaches it. This
clearly makes him feel like James Bond.

A pigeon walks slowly across two roof tiles
of a cottage. He looks around from
this new perspective, and then
ambles back.

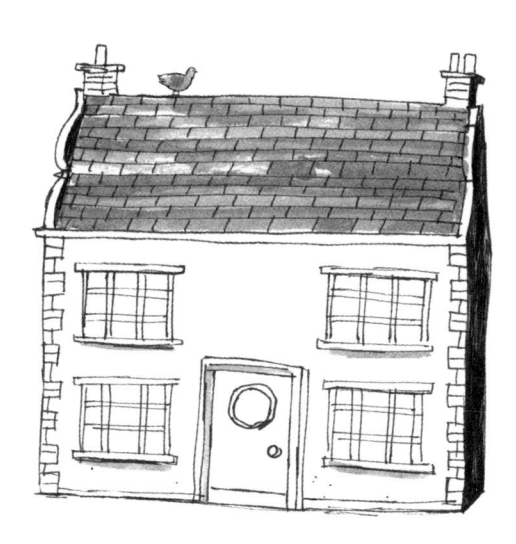

As she walks through this hamlet, a woman's shadow crumples over the cobblestones.

A walk through the forest ends with a frozen lake. Birds walk across the newly solid water with biblical confidence. Tree branches are snow-laden: pure, cold magic.

Two beautiful, brown horses stand side by side in a field. Sun falls across their backs. They are so still they are like paintings of themselves.

Sheep stand on a sunlit farm in Cheddington, Buckinghamshire. The ground is caught between last night's frost and the warmth of the morning. The sheep seem frozen to the spot – perhaps as dazzled by the beauty of it all as I am.

A woman hand-draws a sign outside a pub, adding enchanting, autumn leaves and yellow stars to hold the words in their chalk embrace.

A little girl stops by a flower. She tilts her head, as if listening.
Little girl (calling to her mum): Mum! Flowers wear petals to keep them warm.

AT THE SEASIDE

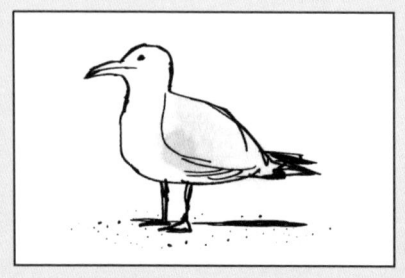

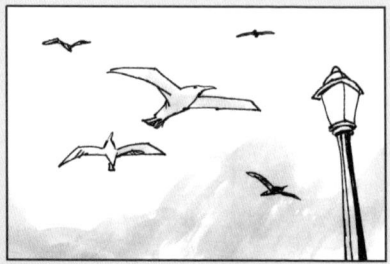

When I'm not there, I'm thinking about it. I was born by the sea and my first home was in a coastal fishing village where the waves constantly threatened to take over. In bad weather they would rush up the high street. When I was very small, I had to be watched continuously because I would walk into the water without stopping, convinced I could breathe under its surface. At night I had tidal wave nightmares. I both fear and love the sea. And I visit whenever I can.

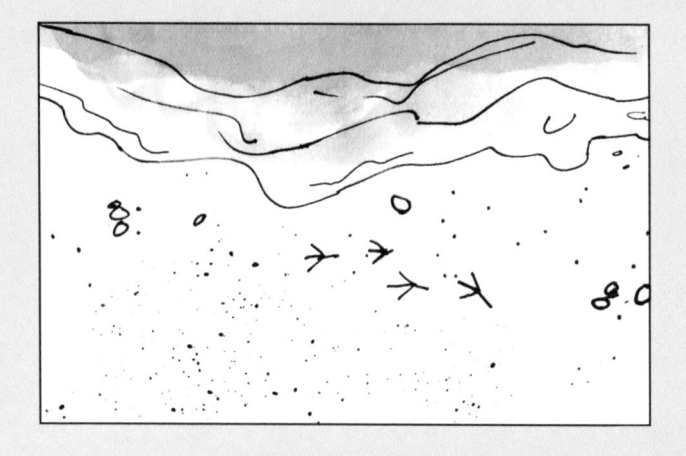

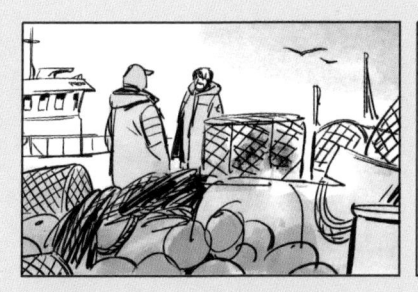

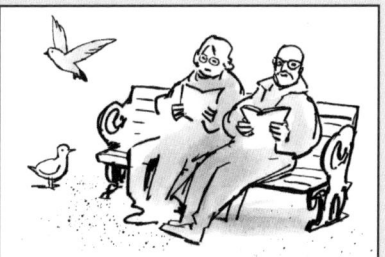

People 'set up home' here, like they do in the park, bringing buckets and spades, sunshades and blankets. And, once they're settled, the sea brings a clarity and focus of its own. Here, even if I'm drawn to a detail for a moment somewhere else, I find myself looking one way: towards the water. My mind slows. I breathe in the salt. I feel the sand between my fingers, the pebbles pushing against my skin. I notice the meeting point between sea and sky.

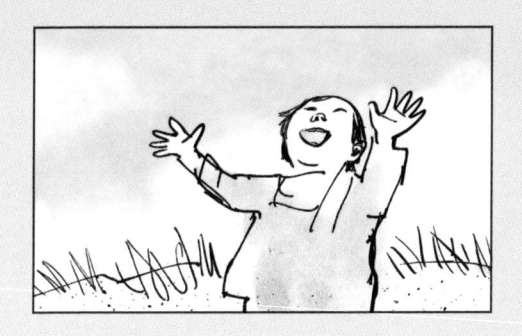

I watch a girl flying a large kite in the shape of a butterfly. In the background, the water is calm and silvery blue. The damp sand is caught mid-ripple from the previous tide.

A woman gets off the bus at Seaham Station
in County Durham. She wears a dark yellow
dress. Its many frills create an echo of sand
from which the sea has just retreated. She
holds a green plant in a wicker-clad pot.
Her dark eyes are small and glittering.

I travel to Southend, Essex, to look at the sea,
but the tide is out until 4:00pm. I will have
to head back to London to pick my daughter
up from school before that. I sit on a wall and
look out across the muddy sand at the thin
band of water in the distance.

A man waves a metal detector over the sand. Beside
him, his teenage daughter uses one too. Hers starts to
make a noise.
The man (to me): I asked her what she wanted for her
birthday: Some new clothes? A trip to Nando's? She said,
'No Dad, I want to look for things, like you.'

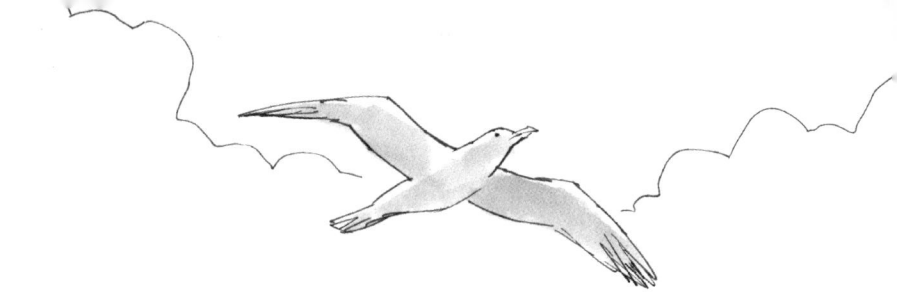

Waves crash against Brighton
Beach, rattling the stones. It is
wild and wonderful. My friend's
swimming costume stays in her bag.

> The sounds of the seaside are very specific.
> The combination of gulls crying, the waves and
> people chatting, playing and splashing relaxes
> me. The noises are the same or similar to those at
> a swimming pool, but how they travel in the open
> is very different. Today, the wind untangles my
> thoughts and pulls at my clothes and hair with
> a refreshing urgency.

Man in Southend: It's too hot here.
I like cemeteries. The best temperature
for a cemetery is 23 degrees.

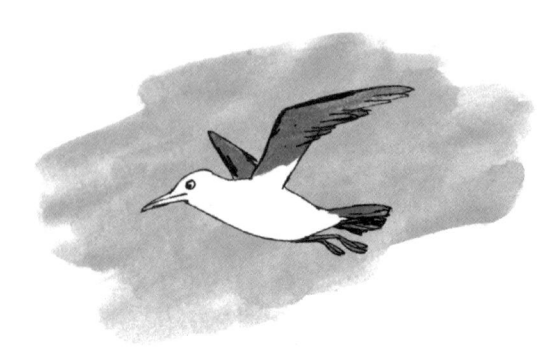

Man in Brighton Station to me as I manage to spill coffee down myself: If the coffee doesn't get you, the seagulls will!

The sun is fierce on my neck and arms. Sand sticks to my feet. A man bounces a baby in and out of the water. His partner photographs them. She looks at the photos on her phone. She says, 'Oh, baby.' The man holds the baby up – his palms support her chest and his fingers curl under her armpits. The baby sticks her legs straight out, and back up behind her – like she is a fishhook. The dad laughs with delight as she performs this surprise circus trick. The woman takes a photo.

A woman in a Mersea Island oyster bar
in Essex studies a copy of the Highway
Code. Moored boats rest just beyond the
window. A bright, orange-red lobster lies
half-dismantled on her plate.

A little girl in Broadstairs, Kent,
has fashioned some splendid new
eyebrows out of wet sand.

A little girl walks across the beach in
Croyde in Devon. The sand has clearly
tried to claim her legs as its own. She
carries a large grey gull feather like
a talisman. Sunlight glitters on
the water.

Children in Hove, near Brighton, make
whooping noises at the waves, inspired by
the water's wonderful energy.

At the seaside

The shadow of a gull passes over my legs. Under my feet, the pebbles are surprisingly comfortable.

A boy with ginger hair bends to pick up a large piece of sea glass and throws it into the sea. He watches it sink. Then he stabs the sharp end of a plastic shovel into the sand so it stands up on its own.

Three men sit talking on a groyne. One of them gets up and wanders away towards the water. He sees something in it. He shouts at the others and gestures for them to come over and have a look. They walk over and wade to where he is standing. All three men look down into the water. I can tell that what they are looking at wasn't what the man had thought it was. He looks briefly embarrassed and then they all burst into laughter and slap each other on the back.

A little boy refuses to get on to the train at Brighton Station until his family agree to refer to him as 'The Most Beautiful of Helens'.

In Chalkwell, Essex, the flat sea glitters. Scattered boats float, almost still. A girl walks, barefoot. Her shoes kicked off behind her for her Nana to pick up.

Woman in a beach café answering her mobile (to what sounds like several people on speakerphone): Afternoon, ladies. [laughs] You been on the Bacardis?

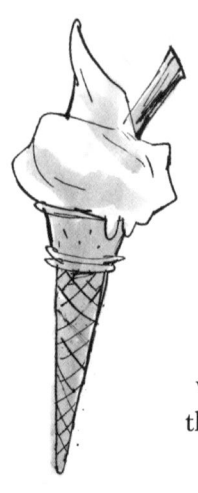

A woman with her husband
begins to count on her fingers:
'It's your choice: fish and chips,
ice-cream or ... no, that's it.'

Even through her mirrored sunglasses,
we can sense that a woman walking along
the pier finds us all rather disappointing.

A person drives through Rye in East Sussex,
drum and bass blasting out of their speakers.
Nearby, people blow on take-away chips
to cool them down and I briefly mistake a
seagull for a statue of one.

A woman plays 'Happy Birthday' on a public piano.
Man: Whose birthday is it?
Woman playing: Someone's.

A child shouts at his scoop of
chocolate ice-cream in a cone.

An optimistic mum tries adult sunglasses on
her baby in a shop. A man feels the weight
of a bucket and spade in his hands. He
goes for a bigger set. A bored shop assistant
behind the counter plays with a bouncy ball
against the till. The air smells of salt.

Man in Ilfracombe, Devon (to his grandson):
What did you like best about the aquarium?
Little boy (after a lot of thought): The fish.

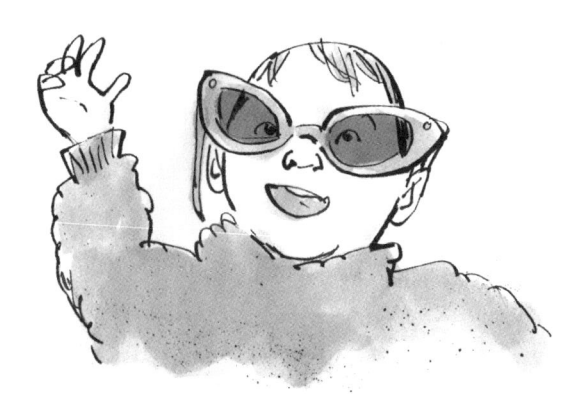

Little girl (looking up at the steel statue of
Verity by Damien Hirst): She's got a sword
and she's about to have a baby. I love her.

A fine mist hangs over Studland Beach in
Dorset, muting the point twixt sea and sky:
the colours of Sunday sugared-almond soft
in the morning light.

A boy stands close to the shallows. He holds
a yellow spade which he uses to scoop up the
pebbles and shells and throw them into the sea.
The tide brings them back again. He repeats.

Two children look for
treasure in the rock
pools. One of them lifts
up a small crab – it grabs
helplessly at the air. She
puts it down onto the
sand. It scuttles away.

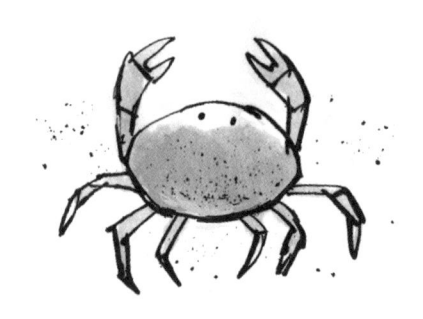

The ocean thunders against the shore in Croyde, Devon. A surfer stands on the sand in her wetsuit facing the weak morning sun, which is losing its battle with the grey cloud cover. It is thrilling to watch the waves slam down – white crests flying across the horizon, but the lifeguards say there will be no swimming today.

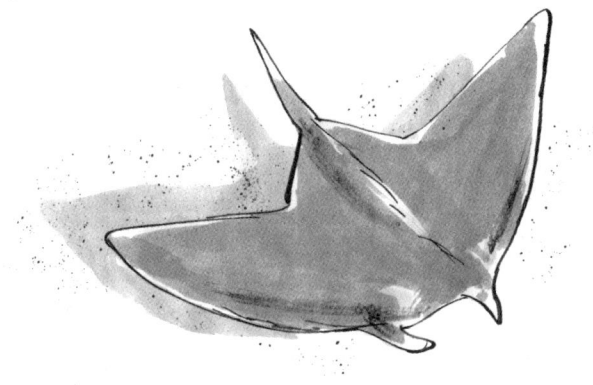

In the Atlantic near La Gomera, Canary Islands, something large brushes my leg. I look under the water – a large ray glides away from me. I feel in awe of its size and grace in the water.

A little boy collects pieces of blue and white pottery that have been worn smooth. He arranges them into a neat circle. He smiles. And then he kicks them into the sea.

At the seaside

Woman walking up the dunes: It's hard, walking up sand.

A toddler in Ramsgate, Kent,
indicates with a sweeping gesture
the beach in general and states, with
confidence, a single word: mine.

Woman outside a beach bar (wearing half
a lobster costume): Yeah, someone ate my
head earlier. In a taco. Ok, I put it down
somewhere. I've lost it. I'm sorry.

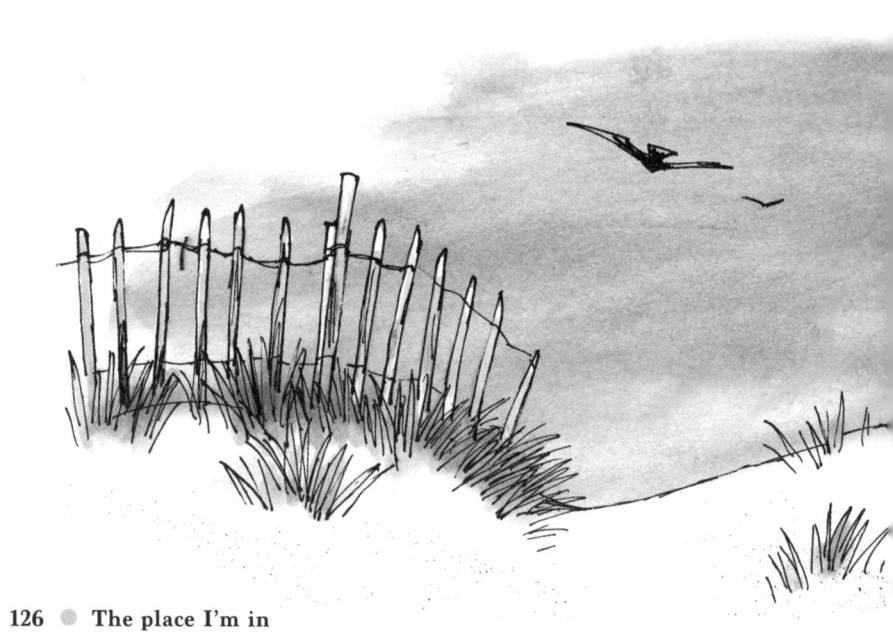

I cycle along a bike path near Woods Hole, Massachusetts. My daughter is in a 'bucket' at the back of the bike, asleep. The sea to my left is blue and the air is clear. I feel lighter than I do in London, like this bike could lift off and fly me over the water.

I pass a sign with information about the planets on it and shout, 'Neptune!' just as a man cycling the other way gives me a look of mild concern. I try to tell him about the planets, but he is gone.

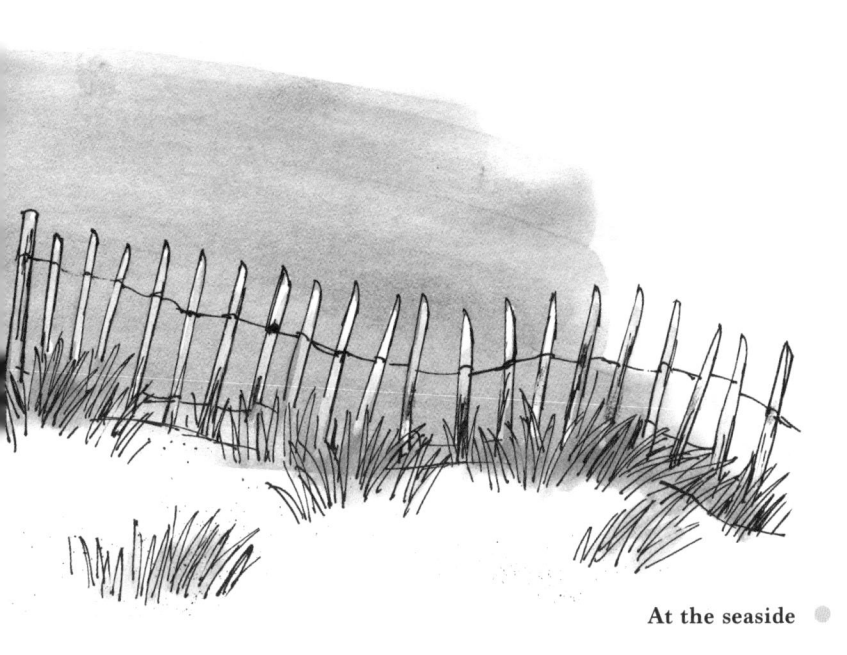

A long way away, a builder knocks
a hammer onto metal. The harbour
carries the sound to make it seem as if
it is happening inside my head.

                  A little girl has spent a while digging a large
                  moat around her sandcastle. She carries sea
                  water in her bucket over to the moat. She pours
                  it in. It disappears. Undeterred, she heads back
                  to get more.

        A woman walks a mesh-sided trolley through
        Winchelsea, East Sussex. Inside are two pugs.
        The woman and I smile at each other.
        Woman: Just taking the old dears to see the sea.

I walk through shallow water by the shore.
Bladder wrack hugs my ankles. Under the water
it wafts upright, with a kind of grace. I bend
down and pick some up out of the sea. It hangs
limply, with that peculiar seaweed smell.

A large blue umbrella escapes the sand – caught by a sudden breeze – and rolls towards the sea. A man carrying a baby runs after it and catches it. He carries the umbrella and the baby back up the beach.

A cloud of suncream wafts over my senses as I pass by a group of parents with their babies in prams – the scent of summer.

Rugby fans at Brighton Station sing en masse and their dense, deep voices swell around us like the incoming tide.

Little girl holding handfuls of seaweed:
I like it. We will put it in the car.
Her mum: No.

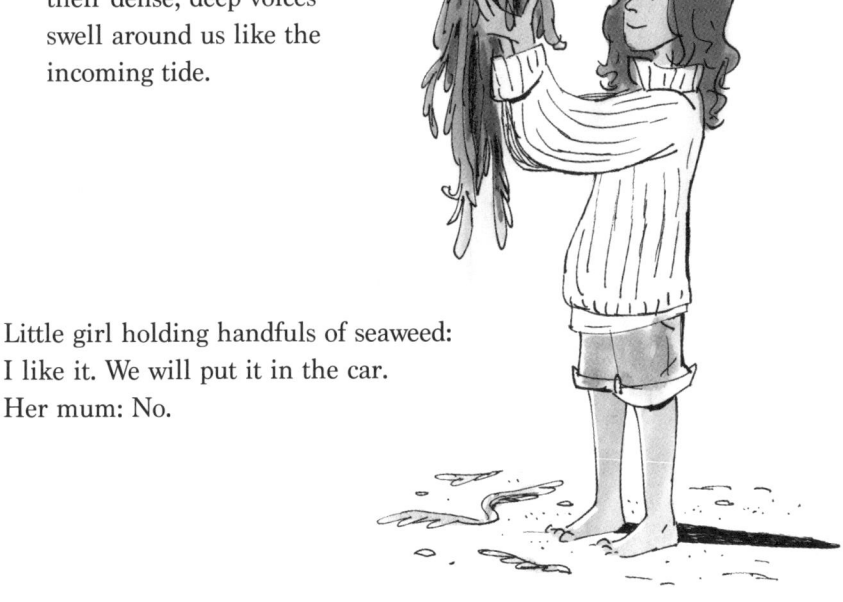

Little girl watching a plane fly over Rye
Harbour, its lights shining through the grey
sky: It's got stars in it.

The tide is out. A gull swoops over the dark,
wet sand towards the shore. An elderly couple
sit on a bench reading paperback novels. A
woman says to herself as she walks past me,
'Wednesday's good.'

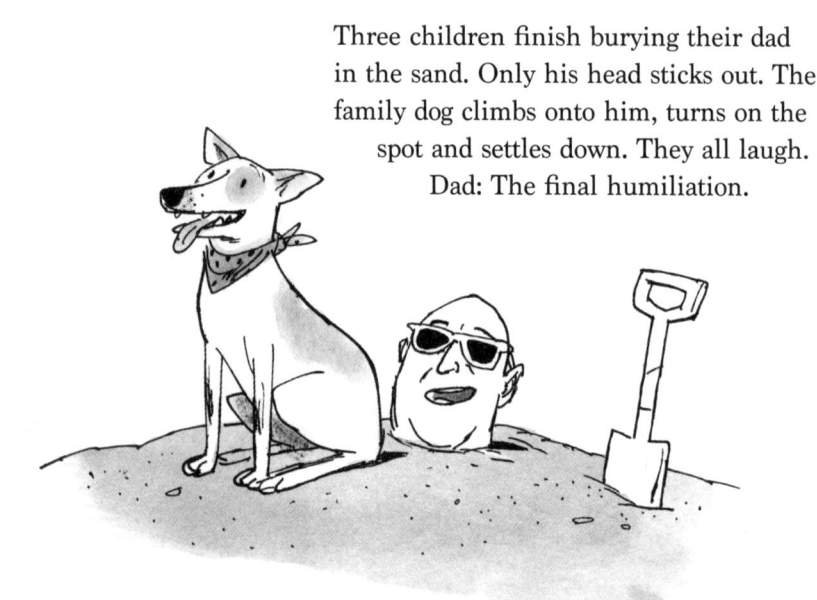

Three children finish burying their dad
in the sand. Only his head sticks out. The
family dog climbs onto him, turns on the
spot and settles down. They all laugh.
Dad: The final humiliation.

A man outside a pub in Blackpool laughs loudly with his friends, a hint of nerves underneath the sound. He is dressed as a bride – this is the start of his stag do.

Two women walk into a seaside restaurant.
A storm wails outside. The women are drenched from head to foot.
Waitress: Get too close to the sea?
They nod.
Waitress: Violent today, isn't she?

A man walks two petite, black dogs in matching coats along the shore, his feet making a pleasing, crunching sound on the pebbles.

ON THE MOVE

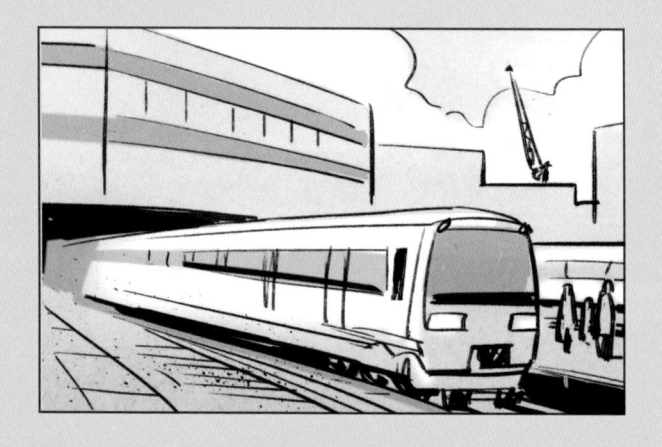

We travel in cars, trains, buses, prams, planes, chairs and bicycles: on foot, on wheels, across water, on rails. We can find ourselves forced together with strangers – their bodies pressing into ours as the tunnels outside the dirty windows rush by dark and close – or sitting alone on the top deck of a bus on a quiet route, where tree branches brush against the windows and the morning sky glows beyond.

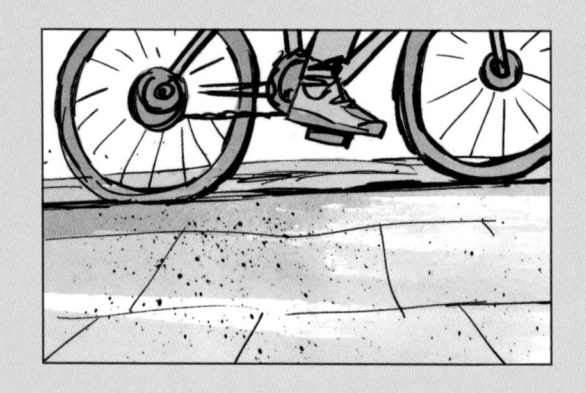

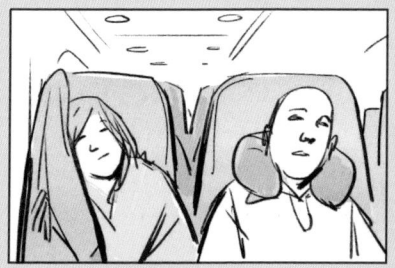

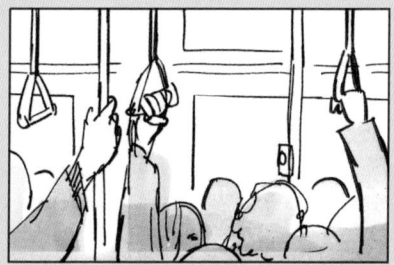

I enjoy noticing how people use their travelling spaces. Some settle in as if they now live here – carefully placing items on the fold-down table to create a makeshift office or living room. Or even a bedroom – folded-up jacket wedged against the window, hand shielding their eyes from the sunlight. There is an odd intimacy in how people nest, folding their limbs into the spaces left by others.

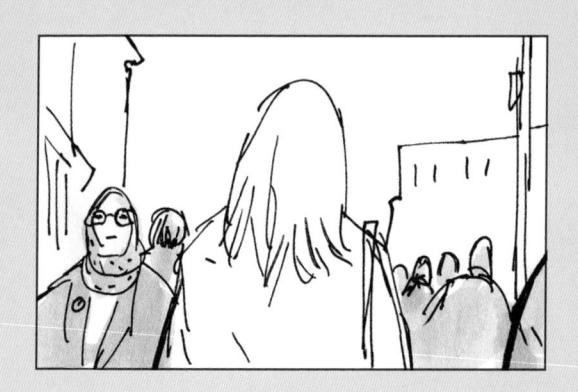

When we arrive at our destination, there's that odd feeling of getting up to move on something that is itself moving – the fight against rocking and lurching that leaves us wrong-footed.

Four teenagers sit together around a table on the
train to Milton Keynes, Buckinghamshire. One of
them takes a tissue out of her pocket and cleans a
small mark from the table. She puts the tissue back
in her pocket. A second girl sprays mousse onto her
hair – the white clouds sit on her head like weather,
before she smoothes them into her ponytail.

> Nearby, an auburn-haired woman sleeps
> behind her hand. Open in front of her is a
> book about pruning trees, the current page
> turned to Silver Birch.

A baby on the train rummages around for
a long time in the depths of her pram seat.
Finally, she finds a small piece of broken
cracker and, with a fabulous smile, she offers
it to the man opposite her.

> Salt on the platform cuts through last night's
> lingering frost.

Little girl (pointing at the carriage ceiling): Aha!
Her mum: Yes?
Little girl: This is a train.
We are on a train.
This is all a train.

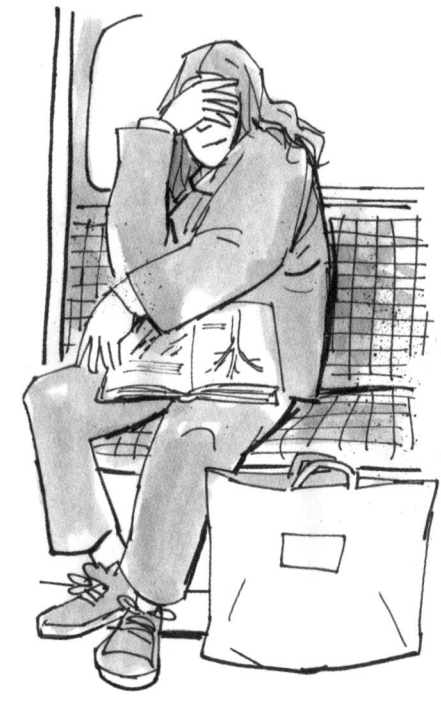

A sudden breeze across the station causes the green, woollen scarf of a man to reach over his shoulder and gently pat his back.

>Man on the train: Would you like this seat?
>Older woman: Thank you.
>She sits down.
>[Pause]
>Little girl: That was nice.

A woman sleeps. As the train sways, the metal buckles of her coat lightly tap her seat with a sweet sound, like distant cowbells.

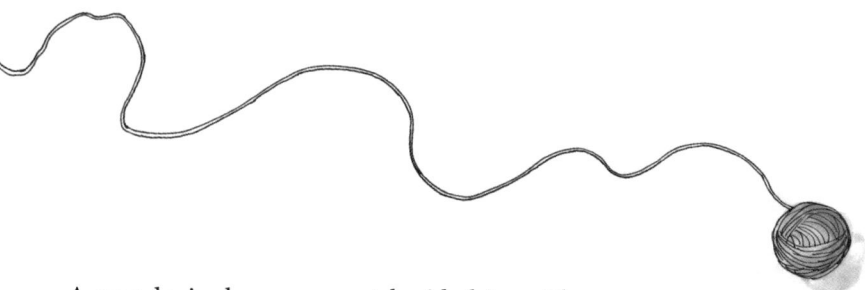

A man lovingly saves a seat beside him with an outspread hand until his final stop. Then with a small sigh, he gets up and off the train.

We stop at Berkhamsted in Hertfordshire. Outside the train, bricks form the surface of the platform. They are arranged like parquet flooring. A train passes in the opposite direction – brief thunder. Trees hunch together in the March light. A woman looks out of the window. She wears a white coat with large white buttons. Her hair is long and dark. She watches something. I follow her gaze. Birds shift and flutter in the tree tops. They are mesmerizing.

A man on the train is asking for change.
He stops near a baby, who gives him a massive smile.
Man (to the baby's mum): Babies always smile at me.
Mum: Maybe they see something good.
Man: Yes. Thank you. I like that.

A woman knits a long, blue and white scarf. Her ball of wool rolls off and under the table and she bends to retrieve it, apologizing to the woman opposite, around whose foot it has become entangled.

I look out of the train window. In the middle of an empty field outside London, someone has made a tower out of rusty old paint cans.

A person gets onto the train holding an
enormous, shiny, pink balloon, and the
wide-eyed little girl next to me whispers
to herself: Oh my days.

The train stops in the tunnel. A man with short,
spiky hair by the door asks, 'Why have we stopped?'
A man nearby, his long hair in a ponytail, tries
an answer, 'Not sure.' There is a pause. He senses
something. 'You ok, buddy?' The man with short,
spiky hair manages an 'Mm hmm.' Ponytail man and
I watch him – wondering the best way to help.
I get up from my seat, to offer it. Ponytail man moves
towards him. Suddenly the train moves. Spiky-haired
man exhales, 'God, I was actually panicking a bit
there, mate. I didn't want to say.' Ponytail man nods.
He says, 'We knew. You're ok.'

Me (to the driver as I get onto
the bus): Morning.
Bus driver (in his turquoise,
mirrored sunglasses): Yo.
We both smile.

A boy films the streets through the window,
rain making everything a blur of colours.

A man walks from the back of the bus to
demist the front window with a tissue.
By the time he gets back to his seat it's
misted over again.

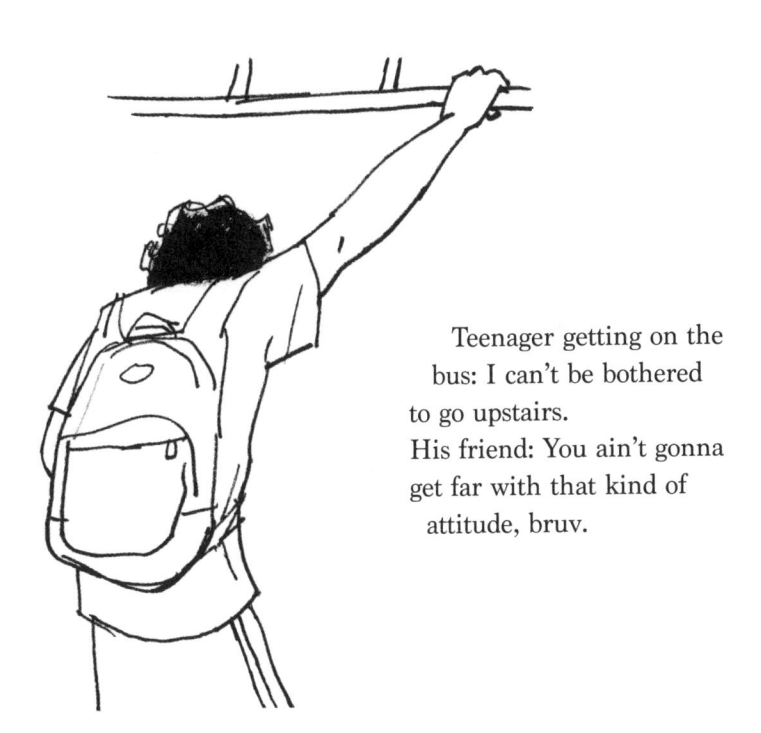

Teenager getting on the
bus: I can't be bothered
to go upstairs.
His friend: You ain't gonna
get far with that kind of
attitude, bruv.

Two men get on, carrying a
coffin-sized cardboard box.
Unnervingly, it is labelled
'Desmond'.

I share an across-the-seats smile with a
mum whose small boy opens and closes
a piece of folded paper, humming as if it
were a tiny accordion.

A man hugs a brown parcel
to himself, forgets he has
it, looks sad, looks down,
discovers it and exhales.

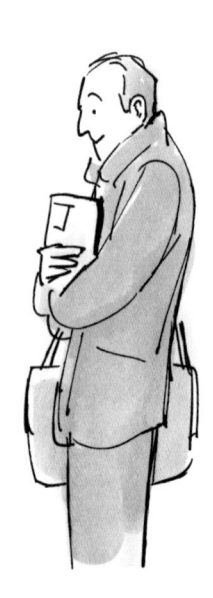

The screen showing the bus's CCTV flicks
through images of its rattling insides, as if
the bus is anxiously trying to diagnose itself.

> A woman walks through Berlin-Tiergarten
> Station and onto the S-Bahn. She wears a
> checked shirt and a yellow rucksack. Her
> green nail varnish matches the green of
> the bookmark that holds a place in her
> paperback book.

From the top deck of the bus, I find myself
suddenly level with a small spider who has
spun a web on a lamppost.

A man drinks up the last of his milkshake through a straw, the sound like a rusty hotel sign swinging in the wind.

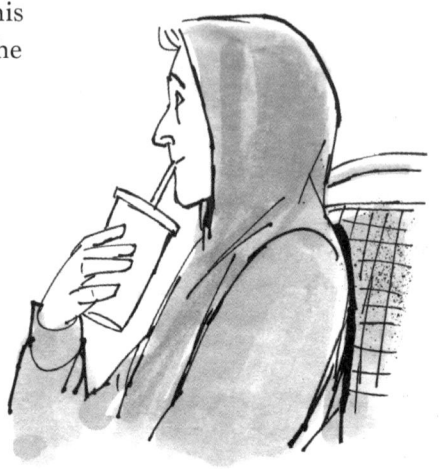

A phone rings on the bus. A white-haired woman opens her voluminous handbag (from which it rings) and shouts, 'I haven't got time for you!' and shuts it again.

As the Tube train arrives at the platform, a man waiting for it gestures with his hand to the carriage door as if giving it permission to open.

Like bees around a flower, rows of high-vis-jacket-wearing schoolchildren swarm into my carriage and past a sleeping woman in a red coat.

A man on the Tube tries to read what I'm writing in my notebook, and I find myself covering the words with my hand.

A fancily dressed woman pretends not to mind as the baby in a pram opposite points at her little, designer dog in his plaid cardigan and shouts, 'Cat!'

Little boy: Ring the bell!
His mum: It's not our stop.
Little boy: Ring it anyway.
His mum: Why?
Little boy: It sounds so nice.

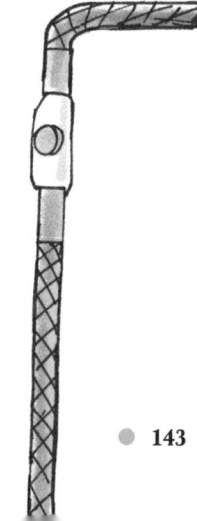

> The rocking movements of this Tube train cause
> the fabric of an empty seat to rise and fall with
> the sighing motion of a sleeper's breath.

A man feels the pulse of a woman.
She waits. Finally she asks, 'Well?'
He replies, 'You definitely have one.'

> A dad sits on a bench on the platform
> with his little girl. It is very warm.
> He looks exhausted. They are
> surrounded by shopping bags.
> She is dressed as a unicorn.

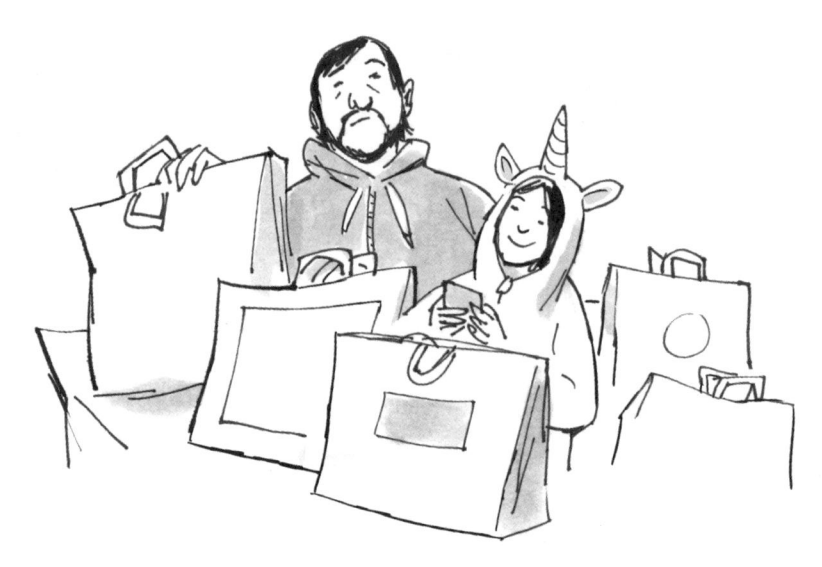

As a woman's umbrella falls towards the Tube floor, incredibly a man catches it with the toe of his shoe and flicks it back up into her waiting hand.

A teenager sits on the Tube, arms folded. He lets out the odd stifled laugh as he tries really hard not to find any of his dad's jokes funny.

A woman on the Tube notices her blue nail-varnish is chipped, searches her bag, finds red varnish, shrugs and uses it to fill in the gaps.

I cycle through the park. In front of me, a man cycles too. The sun makes a sharp shadow of him and his bike on the road. His body and his bicycle become one in shadow, and I feel as though I'm watching a life-sized automaton.

Woman suddenly standing up on the Tube: Oh my God. We're here already.

A man cycles through Clerkenwell, the untethered earflaps from his deerstalker hat flailing fabulously every time he goes over a speed bump.

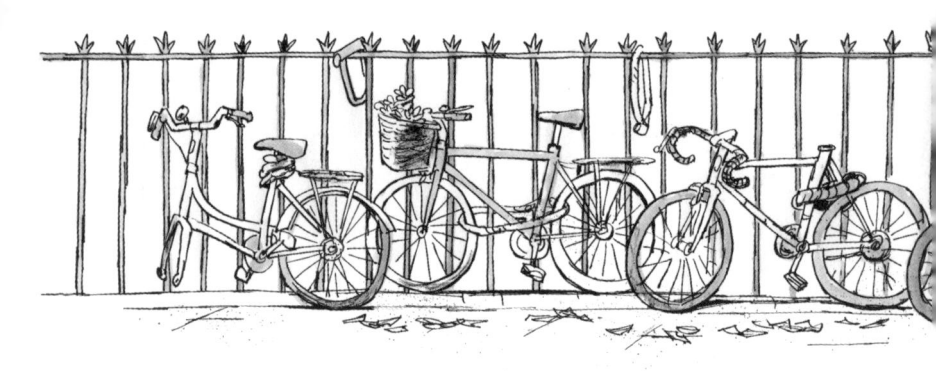

Two men cycle through Old Street in the rain, their increasingly wet Santa costumes sticking to their skin below their happy, damp faces.

A man working on the Thames Clipper ferry carefully lays the thick coils of white rope for docking in a satisfying spiral.

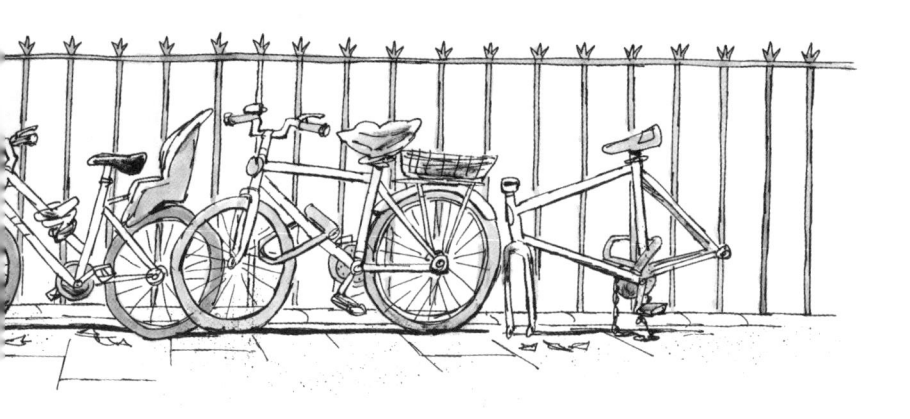

Hail hits me with cold sparks as I walk down the street.

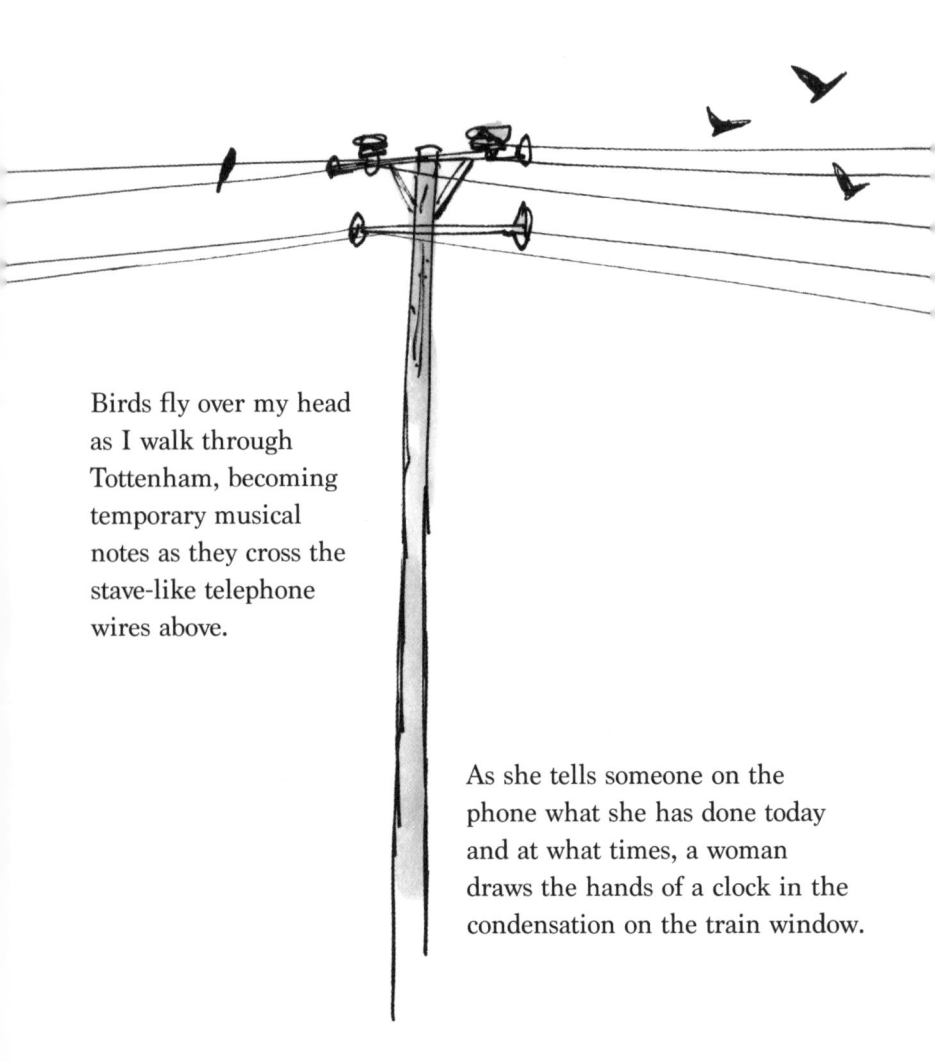

Birds fly over my head as I walk through Tottenham, becoming temporary musical notes as they cross the stave-like telephone wires above.

As she tells someone on the phone what she has done today and at what times, a woman draws the hands of a clock in the condensation on the train window.

A woman crochets a small, round, white, floral-patterned something on the ferry from Gedser in Denmark to Rostock in Germany. The movement of the water beneath us means she sways gently as she does so.

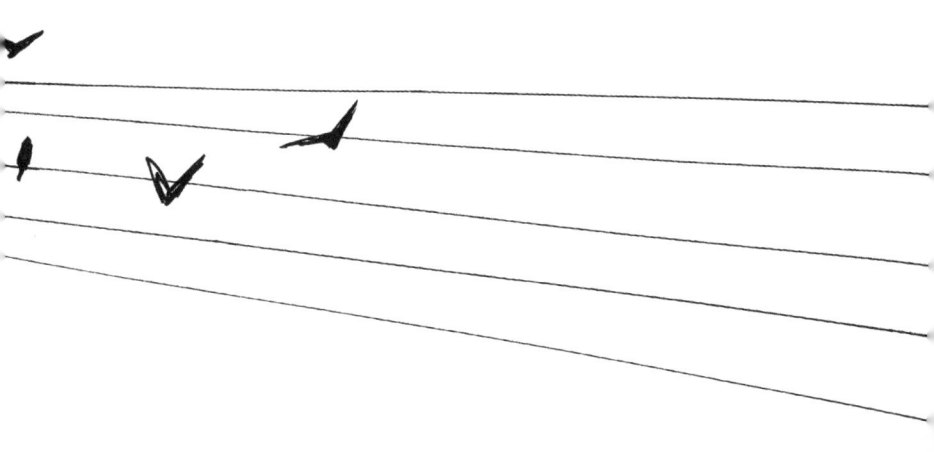

On a florist's stand in New York, many yellow tulips nod their heads 'Hello' as I walk past.

Sun speckles the River Wear as I walk through Durham. Three grey-haired women in a boat row past.

NIGHTLIFE

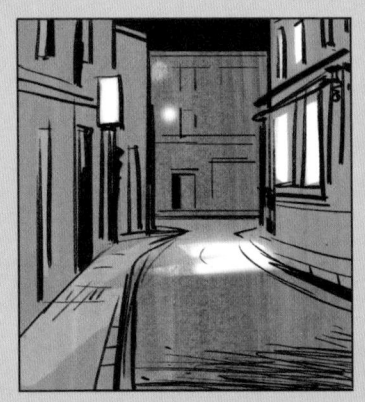

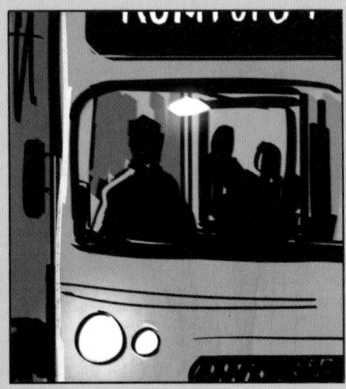

During the day in a city, there is a constant hum of noise. But at night the sound has dramatic peaks and drops. One moment, busy traffic competes with the clamour of a crowded bar. Then, turning onto an empty sidestreet, I hear only my own footsteps.

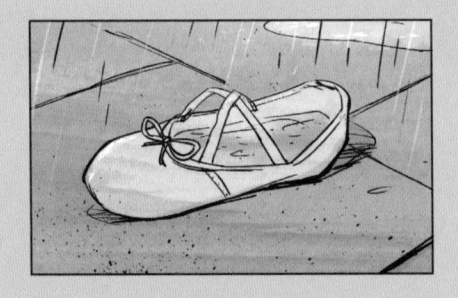

The moments I notice have a distinct feel in the dark. A teddy bear left on a wall in case its owner returns feels somehow sadder when the sun has set. A single ballet shoe filling with rain or the lights of the night bus are given extra significance.

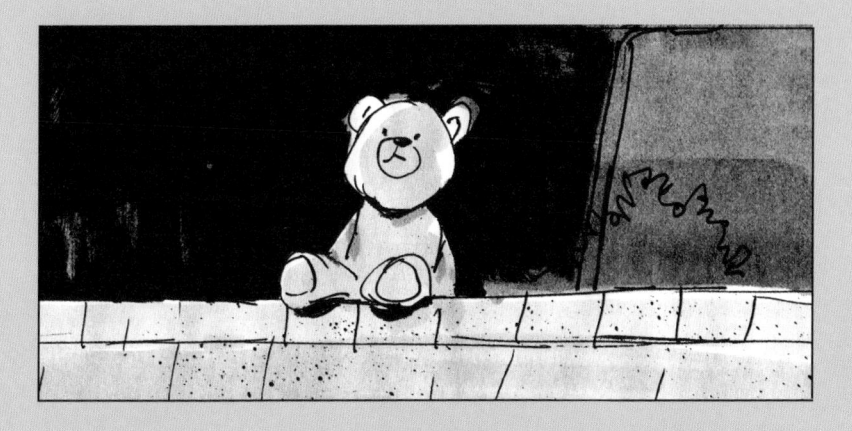

Maybe you notice the white puffs of your breath in the cold air or see that your shadow looms forward and disappears on a loop as you walk under streetlamps. Perhaps a small 'meow' cuts through the silence. Maybe you stop to stroke the cat's tabby head.

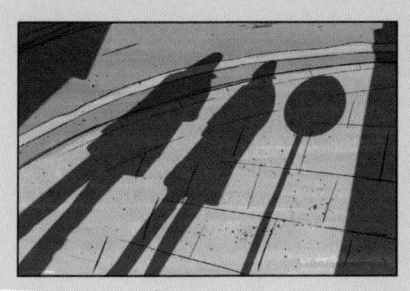

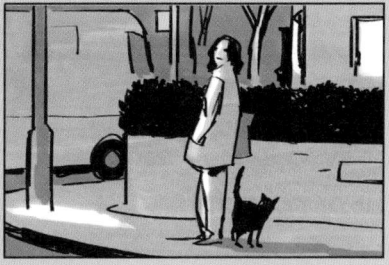

I like long walks, especially at night. They help me think. I used to work late shifts in central London and walk for hours home to Tottenham, arriving at 1am. These days I'm not such a night owl. But I often think about my late walks, and maybe one day I'll get back to them.

Man in a pub: I've not lived in London long.
Woman: What d'you think of it?
Man: It's big, isn't it? I mean, just really, proper big.

Two women laugh as one woman's vodka jelly misses her mouth, and bounces dramatically off her nose to the floor.

Woman (as the first question from tonight's quiz is read out): That next table have a dog. Is that allowed?

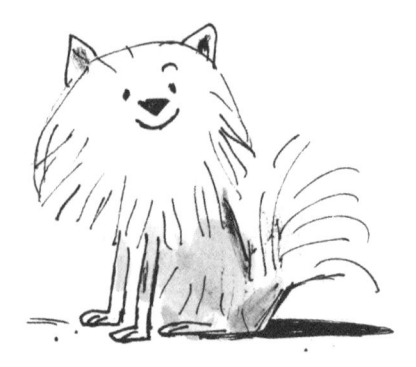

On touching her arm, a man in a bar
realizes the friend he's telling a funny
story is actually asleep behind her hand.

A man in a turquoise-hooded top stares into
his pint as if it contains the world.

Two bar staff flirt outside – the electric
tension between them somewhat confused by
an unwieldy mop that one of them is trying to
hang on to in the wind.

A grey-haired man stands in the pub
garden in old, brown shoes, watching
the rain fall in the dark, a forgotten,
gone-out cigarette in his hand.

On the back of a toilet door in black ink:
I've been coming here for 30 years. The
old door was better.

A woman steps out onto the street,
opens her bag, removes a pair of
trainers, places them side by side on the
pavement, takes off her heels, pushes
her feet into her trainers and sighs.

I walk at the time of night when lights are on
and curtains open. I look into a front room.
It is large – empty, save for a small bed,
the walls coated in a textured wallpaper. A
builder's high-vis jacket hangs from a hook –
half-plaster, half-jacket. Nothing else, but a
dreamcatcher in the window.

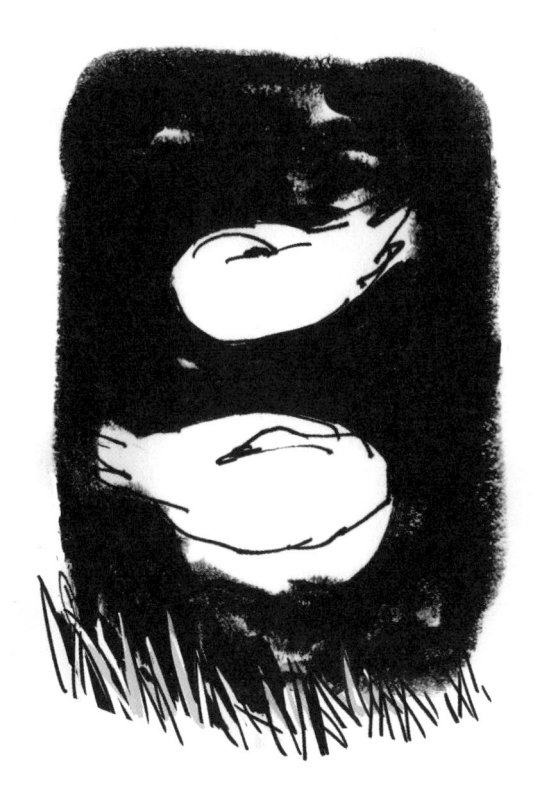

On the windswept canal, the swans sleep, floating in the gathering gloom, their long, white necks curled snugly into their feathered backs.

A paramedic leaving a hospital nods at a colleague who smiles and says, 'Sleep well.'

In a closed-for-the-night supermarket, a single reindeer headband lies face down – its little, red-felt nose squashed against the shop floor.

A woman stands in Euston warily eyeballing her floppy-eared dog, who's definitely decided he wants to spend the entire night on the pavement.

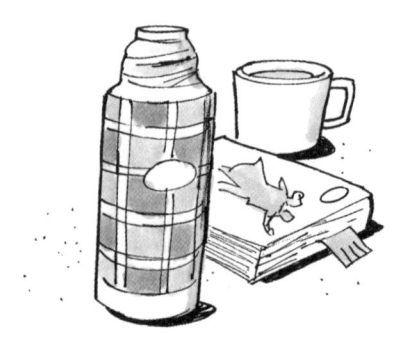

On a late-night train, a woman sits. She drinks from a thermos. She reads a novel with a black-and-white cover of a couple dancing.

Man outside a pub: What d'you make of the new girl?
Woman: The silent one with a weird fringe and a face like thunder?
Man: Yeah.
Woman: I like her.

On the window of the night bus, lit up by the
streetlights outside, is the translucent handprint
of a child, ghostlike against the glass.

I walk past a man on the pavement. Behind
him, a black cat saunters through the dark.
Me: That cat looks like he's with you.
Man: He is.

Two women in matching parkas sleep,
resting their heads on each other's shoulders.

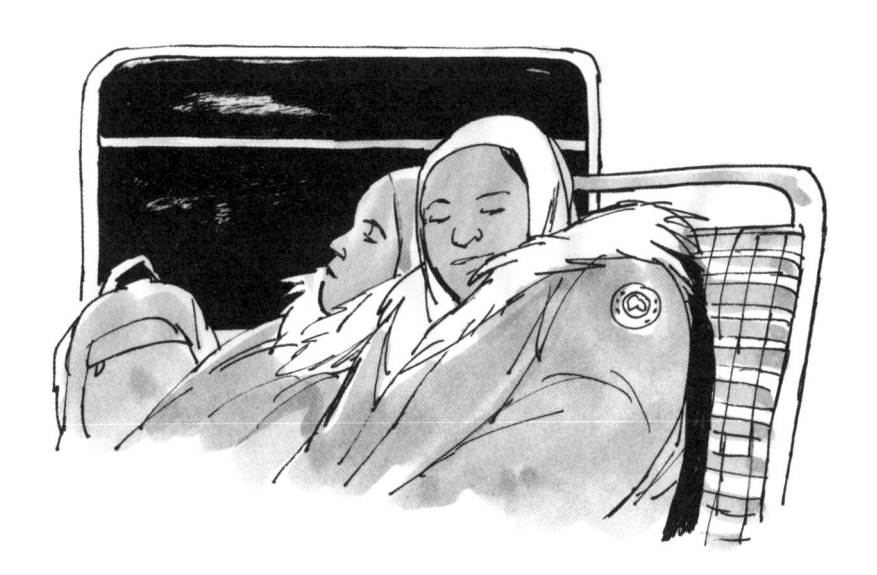

Nightlife

A slightly confused-looking woman in a grey suit stands outside a pub in Greenwich holding a can of Vimto and three large portions of chips.

A man at the window of a house looks out into the darkness as he removes the fairy lights from his tree – winding them around his fingers into a glowing Hulk-hand of Christmas.

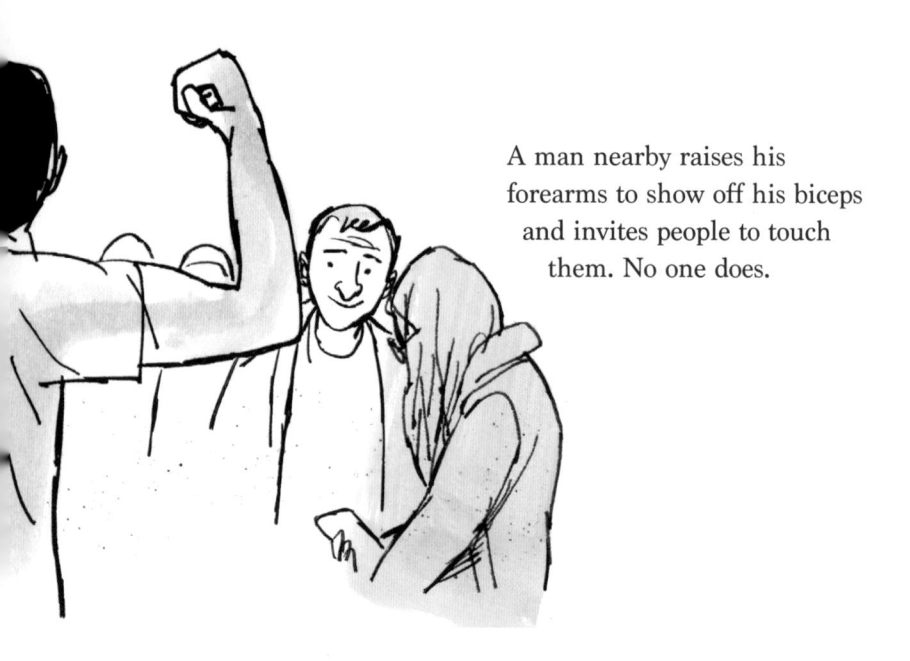

A man nearby raises his forearms to show off his biceps and invites people to touch them. No one does.

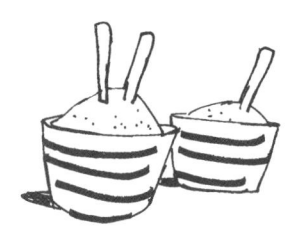

Metal spoons on tables, in a café that is
closed for the night, stand up in bowls of
sugar like newly grown plants out of soil.

A man stands outside a restaurant. He wears a splendid Christmas jumper, the large, glittery penguin embroidered upon it stretching over his Boxing Day belly. Behind him, through the restaurant windows, lights twinkle in the gloom.

On a dark street, two sets of eyes stare at
me from the woollen panda-bear gloves
worn by a woman with long, red hair.

A flock of pigeons rise from behind a wall
in the estate behind me. The beating of their
wings is eerily beautiful on this cold night.

> A man walks through the dark.
> Fading pillow creases decorate his
> cheek, speaking of recent sleep,
> for a night shift to come.

Outside a New Year's Eve party still going strong
stands a man. Muffled music drifts into the air
around him. He is protected from the coming
year by large, orange sunglasses.

> A woman walks through the
> night. Her silver fish earrings
> glitter in the lights – the
> stretching cat on her t-shirt
> destined to never catch them.

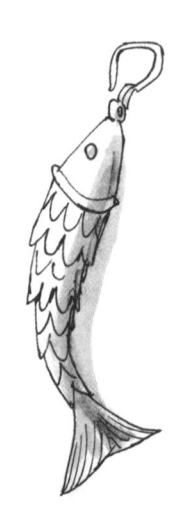

Out of the dark, a leaf falls from a tree. A man wearing a head torch adds it to the pile of leaves he is clearing.

I walk behind a white-haired, barrel-shaped man in denim shorts, his bare legs a surprising sight on this January evening.

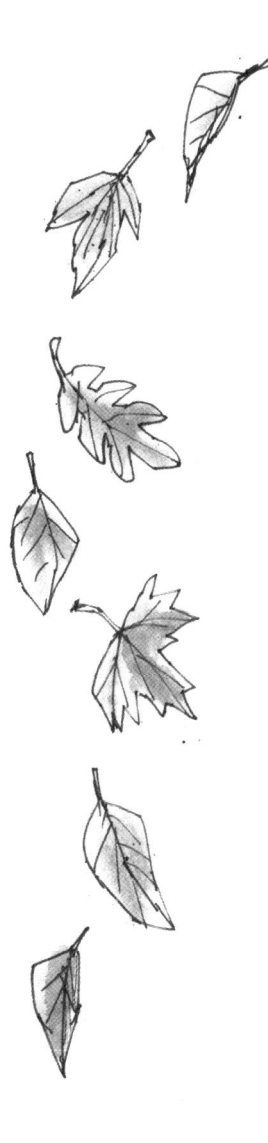

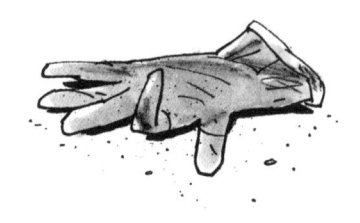

A coincidental shadow-sculpture created by
streetlights and the contents of a skip sprawls
across the pavement with jagged beauty.

A woman in a yellow dress dances with
an imaginary partner outside a betting
shop, a subtle smile on her serene face.

Just as I walk past a house in
Tottenham, someone inside
happens to shout, 'Hooray!',
and it makes me smile.

On a dimly lit street, a black, leather glove lies crushed by the traffic, save for one lifted forefinger, which beckons.

The door of a now-closed gallery opens, and a woman in a pink-feathered turban and a man in a shiny tiara rush into a waiting car.

Many red balloons tethered outside a steakhouse untie themselves somehow and float away into the warm evening sky.

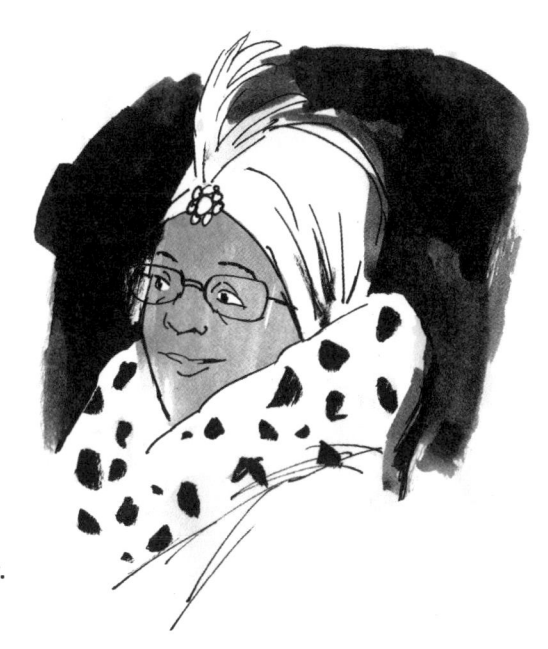

Nightlife

A woman with a white shell clip in
her blue hair gazes at a sand-coloured
dress in the window of a boutique.

A shiny, red notebook lies open and
abandoned, its curly-paged contents now
just inky, watery swirls in the damp air.

A woman by the window of a Turkish
bakery in Hackney tucks freshly made
spinach and feta parcels into their
clingfilm blankets for the night.

A man walks through King's Cross. He wears a broad-brimmed hat. He uses a cane, making small taps as he walks.

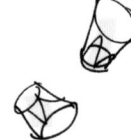

A man sits by the window reading a newspaper in the semi-darkness of a podiatrist in east London.

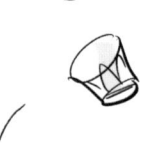

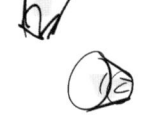

A waiter in a quiet bar throws an empty glass into the air and catches it.

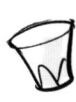

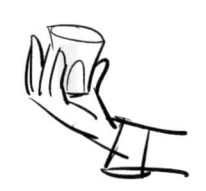

Nightlife ● 165

A woman walks through Walthamstow,
the sequins sewn on her red and gold
sari glowing under the streetlights.

                      A man sits in the waiting room of a vet's
                      with a small terrier on his lap. The man
                      strokes the terrier's ears. Perhaps he has a
                      late-night appointment. Or perhaps he has
                      a date with a vet.

A man plays pool in a pub as disco
lights cast multicoloured circles, like
many sci-fi suns, across his grey hoody.

There is something magical about the
moment in the evening when the solar
lights come on.

A man plays jazz outside on the hot street
– his feet tapping to the molten gold notes
that float from his saxophone into the dark.

From the shadows of an estate, a fox stares at me.
Bold as the brassy tones of its fur, its gaze follows me
unbroken until, suddenly, it turns with a magnificent
swish of its tail and runs off into the night.

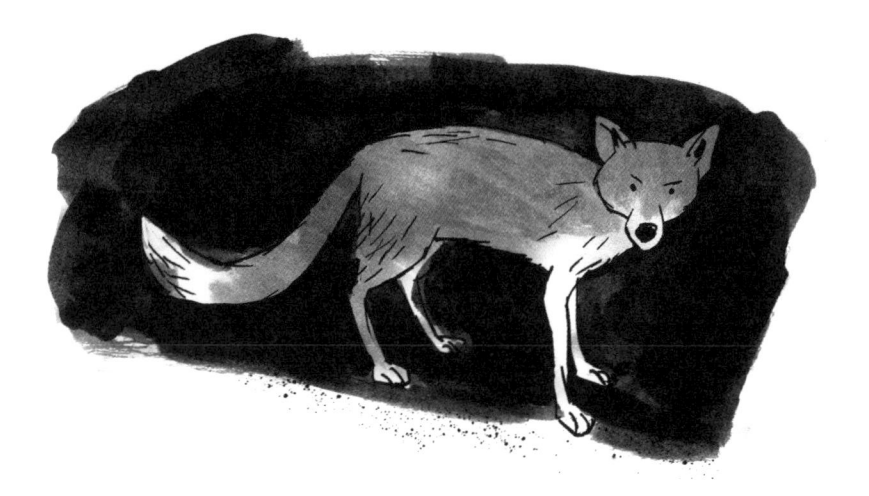

COMING HOME

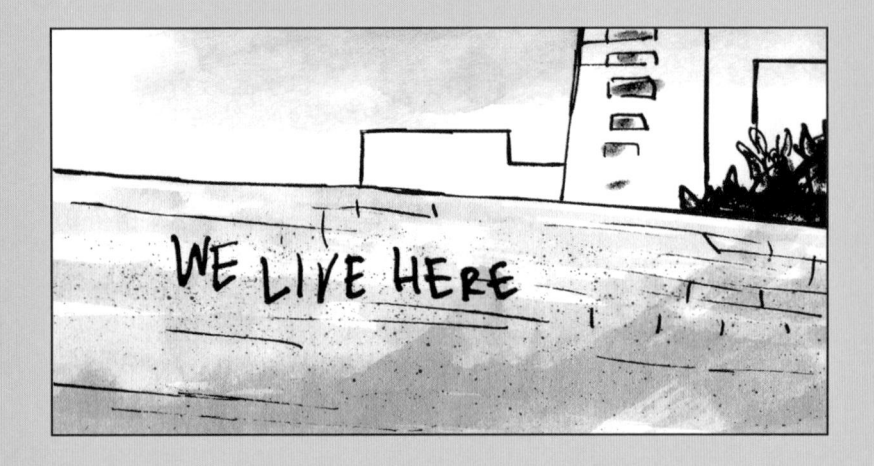

This final chapter's observations were recorded on my way home: after weeks, days, hours or just a few minutes of being away. That feeling of returning that brings a subtle shift of attention is the only thing that connects them.

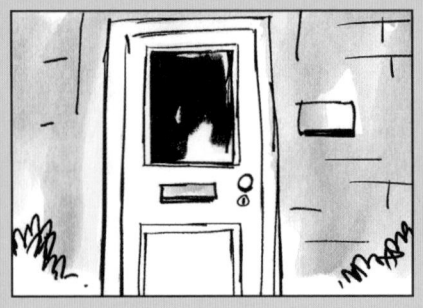

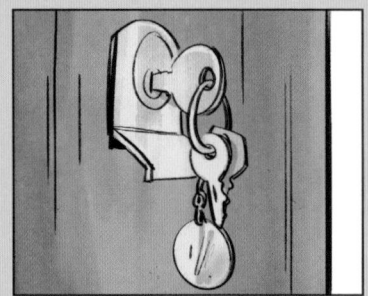

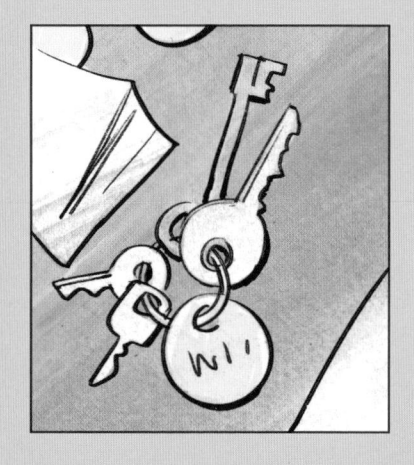

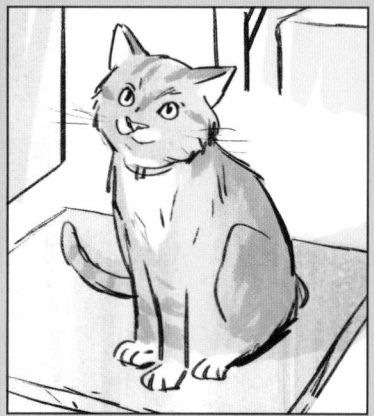

Catching the train or bus that goes to my house, the stops on the way are ones I have looked out at again and again, but have never come home to. Whether I'm returning from the expansiveness of a bustling city or rural landscape, heading home brings a narrowing of focus – an end point. The walk down my street. The sound of my keys. The chirruping-purr of my elderly, tortoiseshell cat as I come in. The familiar click of my front door behind me. The distinctive smell of my house, that I only notice when I've been out of it for a while. Maybe the guilty pleasure of being the only one home. The exhale and small 'hello' as I go to feed the cat.

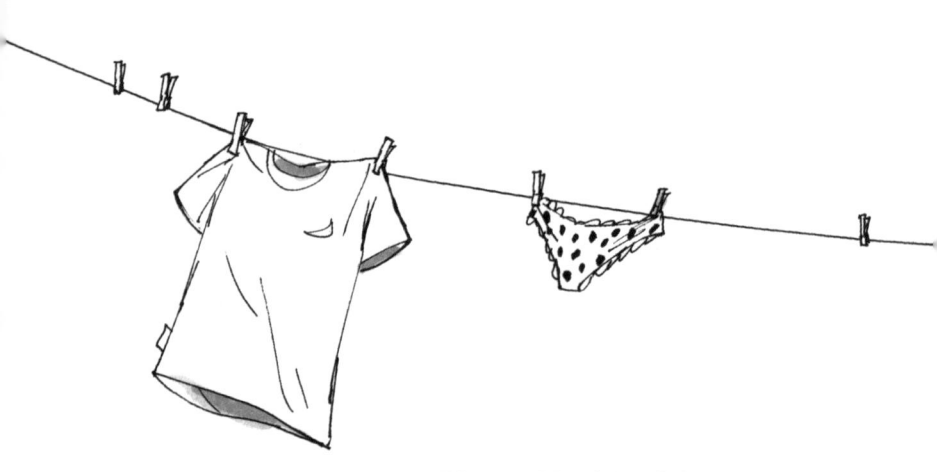

I hear a North Yorkshire accent
behind me on the Tube carriage
and it feels like home – even though
I haven't lived in Yorkshire for what
seems like forever.

A solitary boat follows, with coincidental
precision, a rippling ribbon of orange
city light which is reflected upon the
cold, grey Thames.

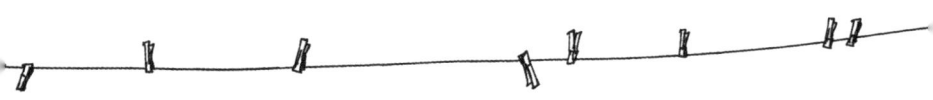

A washing line on the balcony of a block of
flats catches my eye. A tiny pair of red, polka-dot
knickers dances wildly in the wind.

A man pulls a trolley full of shopping
through Dalston – the trolley's rusty,
old wheels screeching like many
hungry seagulls fighting over chips.

A sudden gust creates a constellation of
rose petals as it scatters them from a nearby
bush, over a stormy-sky-coloured car.

A grey pigeon wends its way
across a courtyard, then, with
a flap of its city-encrusted
feathers, lands with tired grace
atop an abandoned microwave.

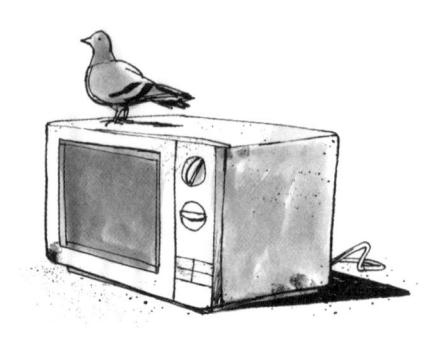

On a desk in an empty office, staple
removers lie on a dark blue file, like
open-mouthed sharks on the surface
of a wintry sea.

As the shadows lengthen, a man in a
dog jumper in an office in Bloomsbury,
his face lit by a computer screen, chews
gum and types.

A busker packs his kit away. His hair falling over his eyes, he settles his guitar in its case, a thought casting a small smile across his face.

A bewildered tourist (as hordes of post-theatre pedestrians rush past him on the Strand): Gosh.

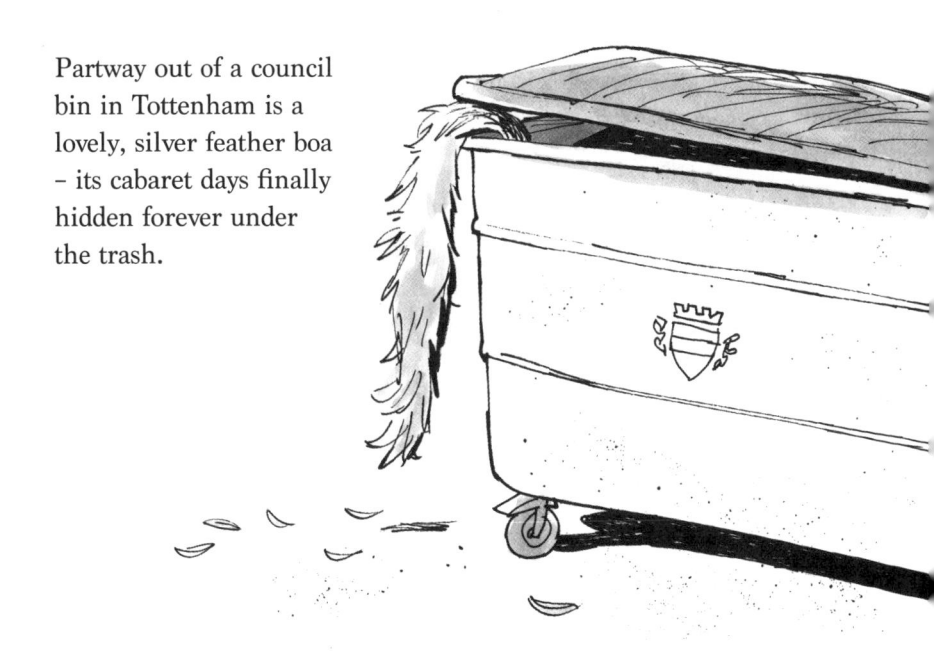

Partway out of a council bin in Tottenham is a lovely, silver feather boa – its cabaret days finally hidden forever under the trash.

On my walk home, I look up to see a large,
arched church window. Back-lit, the dark ribs of
the stairs are in shadow. I wait, half expecting
Nosferatu's silent Count Orlok to charge up them.

A little beetle lands on my screen as
I type on my way home. It walks over
the text as if inspecting it, and, on my
pressing 'send', flies fast away.

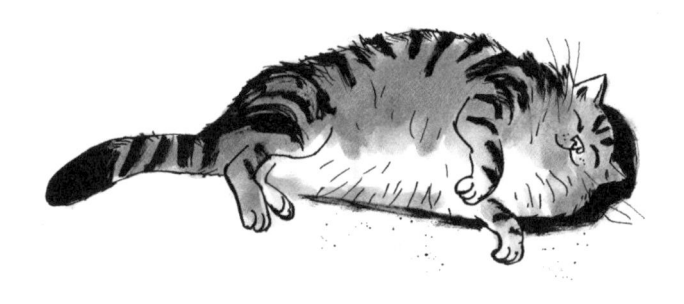

Man on his phone: She's got this cat.
Called Greg. Well, I say cat. He's more
like half-cat, half-sofa.

Woman in Sainsbury's: Where is everyone?
Her boyfriend (sadly): Watching *Doctor Who*.

An old lady and a toddler walk hand in
hand down the road chatting animatedly,
comfortable with each other's natural pace.

Two girls in silver-sequinned cat ears
and drawn-on whiskers dance around a
take-away shop in Crystal Palace as they
wait for their fish and chips.

Rain collects on the face of an old
mirror left on the street.

A telephone engineer works at a junction
box with handwritten notes inside it,
which I secretly hope are love letters from
another engineer.

Little girl making her mum walk around
a leaf on the ground: It's just fallen. It's
exhausted. Give it time to think about it all.

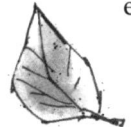

A tailor working late in a suit-maker's
in the city finally decides to head
home, arranging the grey, cashmere
scarf under his coat with expert care.

A tree in town sways in the breeze, as
bright slivers of light from a window
behind burst through its autumn leaves
like pale gold fireworks.

Abandoned mattresses lie on the streets like
beached whales, a forlornness about them, as
they fail to find purpose in this new home.

A bored-looking man in a hat with
bunny ears sits in the window of a tattoo
parlour, practising designs with a Biro on
a fake, plastic arm.

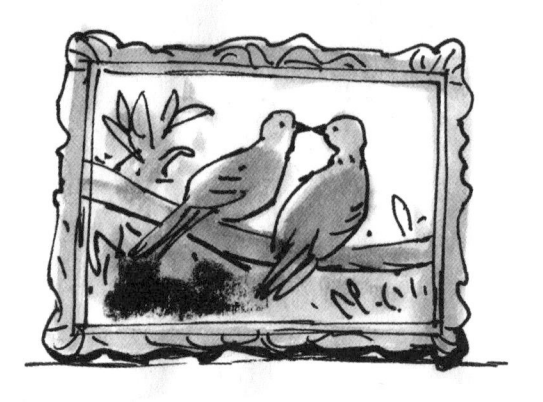

A couple walk along a darkening street.
She pushes a baby in a pram and he
carries a painting of two turtle doves.

Two smartly dressed women with perfect
hair wait to cross the road, each with
their left foot lightly resting on a scooter.

Two giggling, bearded men sit together
in Old Street, listening to a rapid,
high, squeaky Italian voice playing
loudly on a cassette Walkman.

With hand gestures as gracefully swooping as birds
in flight, a man working in a busy off-licence
describes a bottle of wine to a customer.

A waitress at the back of a quiet,
Vietnamese restaurant in east London
eats tangles of rice noodles with an
elegant command of chopsticks.

Two men struggling to fit an old, leather
sofa through a doorway are taking the
radical step of sawing off one of its legs.

I've got 'Let It Be' by the
Beatles stuck in my head. As life
philosophies go, it's not a bad one.

Outside the Rio Cinema, a girl in a grey cardigan smokes a roll-up and stares thoughtfully at the tide-like rhythms of the passing crowds.

Man leaving the cinema: It had no plot and was entirely unconvincing. And I didn't like a single character. That's life I guess.

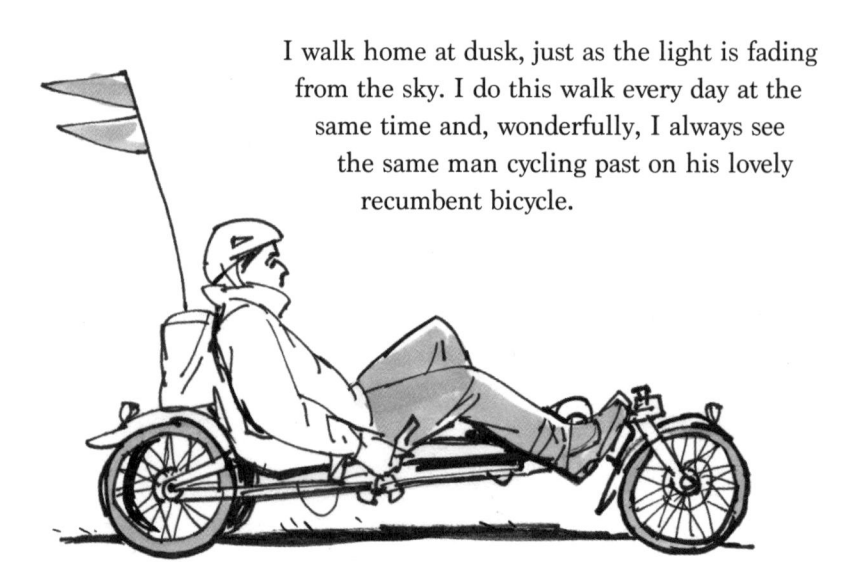

I walk home at dusk, just as the light is fading from the sky. I do this walk every day at the same time and, wonderfully, I always see the same man cycling past on his lovely recumbent bicycle.

An elderly man walks along
the Southbank in the damp air,
singing Elvis songs softly to
himself in a rich-as-treacle voice.

                              A man closes the doors at the back of his van,
                              plunging into darkness the glimmering rows
                              of red, sparkly dresses inside.

A tiny, brown dog in a tiny, corduroy coat, with
a tiny, daffodil brooch pinned to its tiny collar,
waits patiently outside a shop for its owner.

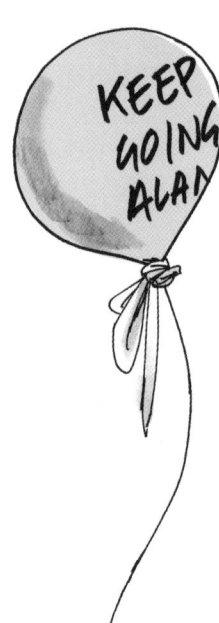

A man in Tottenham stands
by a hatchback contemplating
steam pouring from its engine,
as a cream-coloured moon rises
behind him in an indigo sky.

A pair of slightly broken, pale pink,
ceramic wellington boots lean into each
other on the pavement, glimmering softly
under a streetlight.

Into my garden from somewhere
nearby floats a red balloon, on which
someone has written in permanent
marker, 'Keep going Alan'.

Woman opening her front door (to the person standing on the doorstep): It's all very well saying you were waiting outside my house for ages. You didn't ring the doorbell. What am I, psychic?

Like a friendly cat, a single, mustard-coloured, autumn leaf follows me part of my way home, carried upon a late September breeze.

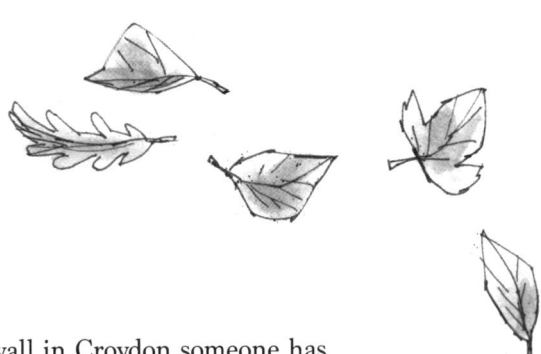

On a brick wall in Croydon someone has written, 'We live here'.

A bemused mum in Clerkenwell watches as her little
girl turns to her schoolfriends as they reach her
house and says, 'Ladies! Kindly remove your hats.'

A huge, black cloud gathers above an office
building with such intense focus, it has
clearly been asked to rain on it specifically.

A slim woman in a long, black coat
tightly wraps her lilac-gloved hands
around herself, as if trying to stop
something from escaping.

Me to my neighbour's builder as he packs
up for the day: You've got such a similar
voice to the guy who came yesterday.
Were you born in the same place?
Builder (laughing): Yes. Our mum.

A tiny, elderly lady rings my doorbell.
I answer.
Her: You are Portuguese?
Me: No.
Her: You speak Portuguese?
Me: No.
Her: Ah, so sad for you.

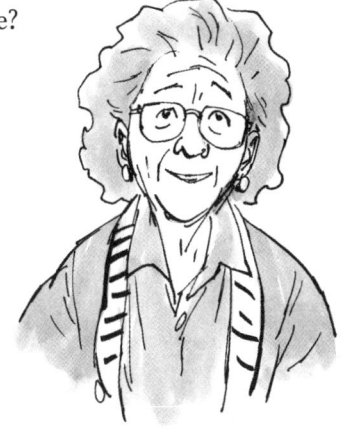

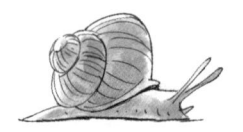

I gently pick up a snail and settle it
on my palm and, unsurprised as I
am, I still find myself in awe, as from
the smooth, grey surface suddenly
protrude two eye-ended tentacles to
tentatively look around.

Just visible in the lit square of an open window
in the house behind mine, a child's dress, the
colour of faded yellow roses, dances in the air.

Night has fallen. Outside my house,
men walk back home from the
mosque. Inside, my cat purrs from
behind me on the back of the sofa.
Then, small noises as she prepares
her paw for cleaning her ears.

As she tries to fall asleep, my daughter asks me to sing her a lullaby. I want to freeze this moment in time – old enough to ask for a lullaby, to know the word, and young enough to want one. I begin to sing. In seconds, she sleeps. I finish the song softly and head downstairs

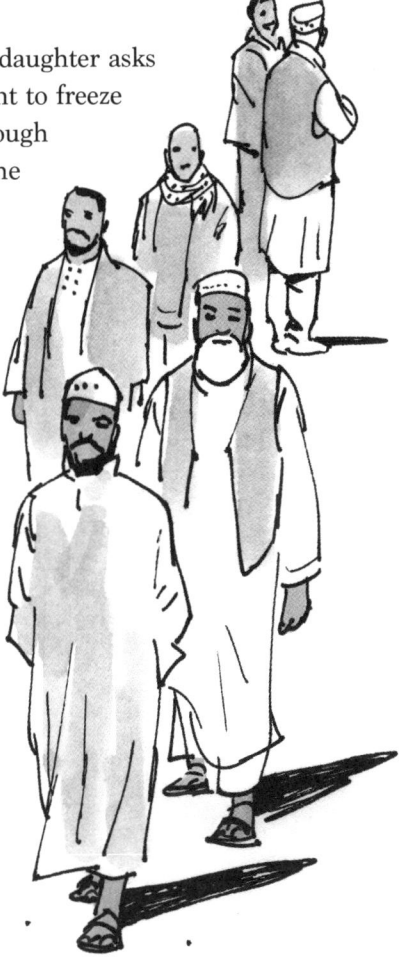

188 ● The Place I'm In

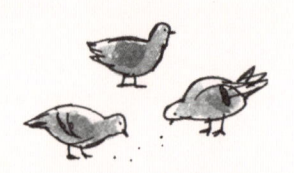

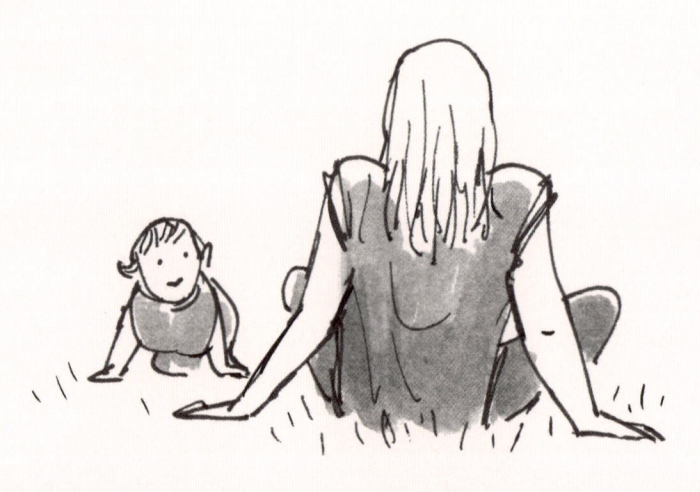

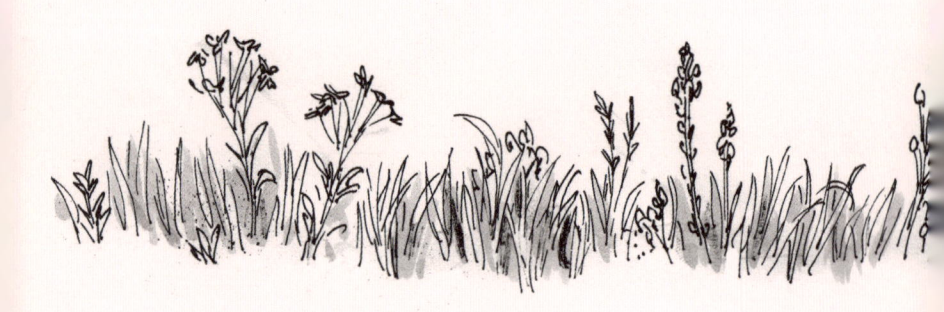

ACKNOWLEDGEMENTS

A huge thank you to my wonderful editor Sophie Lazar, who always believed in this book and who made it the best it could be. I loved our conversations about the details we notice, and mazes and dinosaurs and everything else in between. Thank you to my brilliant agent Anna Power of Johnson and Alcock. I wouldn't have got this far without your sharp and creative mind helping to hone my collection of ideas into something solid. A huge thank you goes to Adam Beer for somehow climbing right inside my head and drawing his perfect take on what he saw in there. Thank you to Duncan McMillan for your thoughts and encouragement and to Bea for being the best. Thank you to Ceinwen McMillan and Ceri Ashcroft for your sharp eyes and kind words. Thank you to Philip Pullman for your encouragement once again – it means the world. Thank you to Ian McMillan for always supporting my writing and for helping me to believe in it. Thank you to everyone at Quarto. The vast majority of this book has been made possible by all the libraries, galleries, museums, parks and public spaces that are free and available to explore, so thank you to all the places I visited along the way. And finally, to my elderly cat Maple, who sat on my words whenever she could, to ensure that I stop writing and stroke her instead.

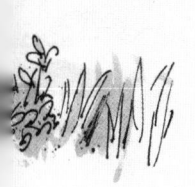

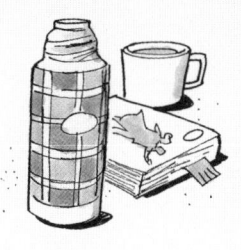

ABOUT THE AUTHOR

Miranda Keeling is a writer, performer and presenter. She writes plays, screenplays, short stories, articles, podcasts and poems. As an actor she works in radio, voiceover, TV, film and stage and is a winner of the BBC Norman Beaton Fellowship. She is the author of *The Year I Stopped to Notice*. She lives in London.

ABOUT THE ILLUSTRATOR

Adam Beer has been working as a freelance storyboard artist and illustrator for over twenty years. He illustrated the picture books *Mammoth* (2021) and *Moggie McFlea* (2024) and wrote and illustrated *Solo* (2022). He has an MA in children's illustration and was shortlisted for the Klaus Flugge Picture-book Prize in 2022. He likes nothing better than strolling around town with a sketchbook and a pocketful of pens.

About the author   191

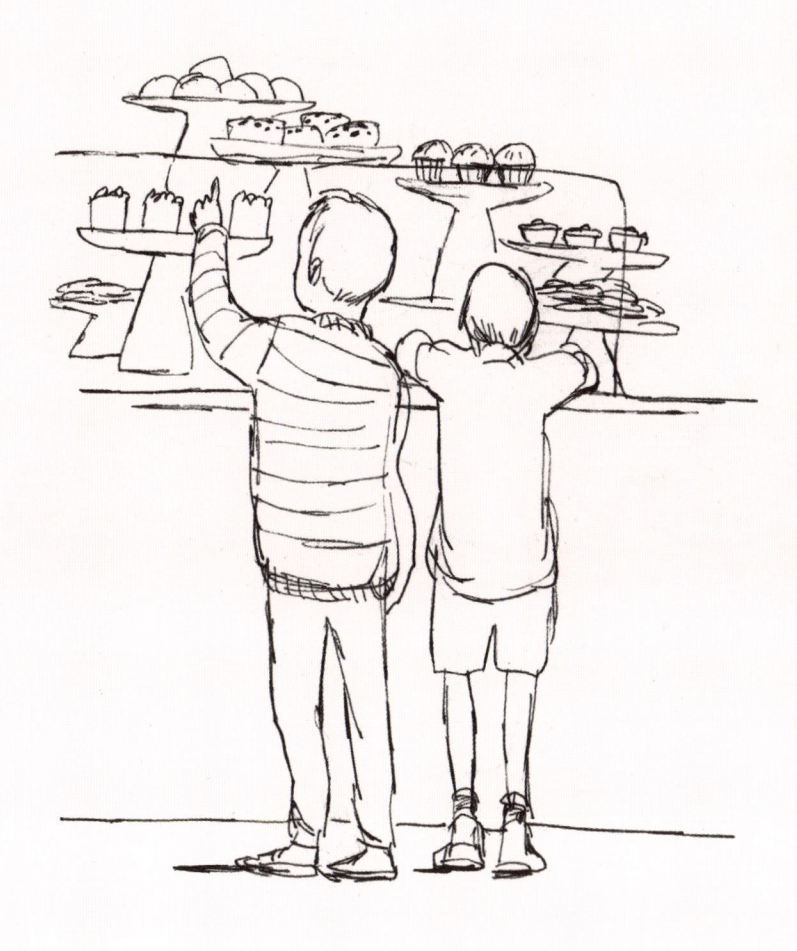

Quarto

First published in 2025 by Leaping Hare Press
an imprint of The Quarto Group.
One Triptych Place, London, SE1 9SH, United Kingdom
T (0)20 7700 9000
www.Quarto.com

EEA Representation, WTS Tax d.o.o., Žanova ulica 3, 4000 Kranj, Slovenia

Text © 2025 Miranda Keeling
Illustrations © 2025 Adam Beer
Design © 2025 Quarto Publishing Plc

Miranda Keeling and Adam Beer have asserted their moral right to be identified as the Author and Illustrator of this Work in accordance with the Copyright Designs and Patents Act 1988.

All rights reserved. No part of this book may be reproduced or utilised in any form or by any means, electronic or mechanical, including photocopying, recording or by any information storage and retrieval system, without permission in writing from Leaping Hare Press.

Every effort has been made to trace the copyright holders of material quoted in this book. If application is made in writing to the publisher, any omissions will be included in future editions.

A catalogue record for this book is available from the British Library.

ISBN 978-1-83600-479-0
EBOOK ISBN 978-1-83600-480-6

10 9 8 7 6 5 4 3 2 1

Book Designer: Nicki Davis
Commissioning Editor: Sophie Lazar
Editorial Director: Jenny Barr
Publisher: Monica Perdoni
Senior Designer: Renata Latipova
Senior Production Controller: Rohana Yusof

Printed in China

MIX
Paper | Supporting responsible forestry
FSC® C016973